VAGUS NERVE STIMULATION
SECOND EDITION

Cover artwork by Simon Powell, an English artist with epilepsy

VAGUS NERVE STIMULATION
Second edition

Edited by

Steven C Schachter MD
Associate Professor of Neurology
Harvard Medical School,
Director of Research
Department of Neurology
Beth Israel Deaconess Medical Center
Boston MA
USA

Dieter Schmidt MD
Emeritus Professor of Neurology
Epilepsy Research Group
Free University of Berlin
Berlin
Germany

informa
healthcare

New York London

Supplementary Resources Disclaimer

Additional resources were previously made available for this title on CD. However, as CD have become a less accessible format, all resources have been moved to a more convenient online download option.

You can find these resources available here: https://www.routledge.com/9781841842578

Please note: Where this title mentions the associated disc, please use the downloadable resources instead.

First published in 2003 by Martin Dunitz, an imprint of Taylor & Francis.

This edition published in 2011 by Informa Healthcare, Telephone House, 69-77 Paul Street, London EC2A 4LQ, UK.

Simultaneously published in the USA by Informa Healthcare, 52 Vanderbilt Avenue, 7th Floor, New York, NY 10017, USA.

Informa Healthcare is a trading division of Informa UK Ltd. Registered Office: 37–41 Mortimer Street, London W1T 3JH, UK. Registered in England and Wales number 1072954.

©2011 Informa Healthcare, except as otherwise indicated

No claim to original U.S. Government works

A CIP record for this book is available from the British Library.

Library of Congress Cataloging-in-Publication Data available on application

ISBN-13: 9781841842578

Contents

Contributors

Berry Anderson RN
Clinical Research Nurse
Medical University of South Carolina (MUSC)
Charleston SC
USA

Daryl E Bohning PhD
Professor of Radiology
Medical University of South Carolina (MUSC)
Charleston SC
USA

Jeong-Ho Chae MD
Visiting Research Scientist
Medical University of South Carolina (MUSC)
Charleston SC
USA
Assistant Professor of Psychiatry
Catholic University, Seoul, Korea

Mark S George MD
Distinguished Professor of Psychiatry, Radiology, and
Neurology,
Director of the Brain Stimulation Laboratory (BSL) and the
Center for Advanced Imaging Research (CAIR)
Medical University of South Carolina (MUSC)
Charleston SC
USA

Christi N Heck MD
Assistant Professor of Neurology
USC Keck School of Medicine
Los Angeles CA
USA

Thomas R Henry MD
Associate Professor of Neurology
Director, Emory Epilepsy Center
Department of Neurology
Emory University School of Medicine
Atlanta GA
USA

Andras A Kemeny FRCS (MD)
Consultant Neurosurgeon
Royal Hallamshire Hospital
Sheffield
UK

F Andrew Kozel MD
Instructor in Psychiatry and Research Imaging
Fellow
Medical University of South Carolina
(MUSC)
Charleston SC
USA

Marina Kurian MD
Department of Surgery
Lenox Hill Hospital
New York NY
USA

Xiangbao Li MD
Visiting Research Scientist
Medical University of South Carolina
(MUSC)
Charleston SC
USA

Qiwen Mu MD PhD
Visiting Research Scientist
Medical University of South Carolina
(MUSC)
Charleston SC
USA

Ziad Nahas MD
Assistant Professor of Psychiatry
Medical University of South Carolina
(MUSC)
Charleston SC
USA

Mitchell Roslin MD FACS
Department of Surgery
Lenox Hill Hospital
New York NY
USA

A John Rush MD
Professor & Vice-Chairman for Research
Department of Psychiatry
University of Texas Southwestern Medical
Center
Dallas TX
USA

Steven C Schachter MD
Associate Professor of Neurology
Harvard Medical School
Director of Research
Beth Israel Deaconess Medical Center
Boston MA
USA

Dieter Schmidt MD
Emeritus Professor of Neurology
Epilepsy Research Group
Free University of Berlin
Berlin
Germany

Foreword

The approval of the VNS Therapy System™ (Cyberonics Inc.), formerly known as the Neuro Cybernetic Prosthesis by the Food and Drug Administration in 1997 'for use as an adjunctive therapy in reducing the frequency of seizures in adults and adolescents over 12 years of age with partial seizures which are refractory to antiepileptic medications' and the earlier approval in Europe were watershed events in the history of seizure therapy. Vagus nerve stimulation (VNS) was the first – and remains the only – non-pharmacological treatment developed, tested in several randomized controlled trials, and approved for epilepsy.

Now more than five years after FDA approval, over 17,000 patients with epilepsy worldwide have been treated with VNS Therapy. This second edition presents the scientific aspects of VNS and details recent advances in the understanding and application of VNS Therapy for epilepsy and other conditions.

The first chapter discusses the theoretical basis of VNS for epilepsy, the physiological effects of vagus stimulation in animals and humans, and the results of acute and chronic VNS in animal seizure models. Chapter 2 reviews the technical aspects of surgical implantation of the VNS Therapy System. Actual video footage from an implantation procedure with explanatory commentary may be found on the CD-ROM that accompanies this book. Chapter 3 presents the efficacy, safety, and tolerability of VNS in clinical epilepsy studies. Chapter 4 outlines the theoretical basis of VNS for the treatment of depression and Chapter 5 presents the clinical trial results of VNS Therapy for depression. Chapter 6 highlights the potential use of VNS Therapy for obesity. The place of VNS Therapy in the current treatment of epilepsy is the subject of Chapter 7. The final chapter provides practical advice for physicians who treat patients with VNS and numerous answers to commonly asked questions. The CD-ROM also contains a comprehensive bibilography of VNS-related references as well as the current Physican's Manual.

As with the first edition, our hope is that this book will foster interest and further development of VNS Therapy.

Steven C Schachter, MD
Dieter Schmidt, MD

Vagus nerve stimulation for epilepsy: anatomical, experimental and mechanistic investigations

Thomas R Henry

1

Introduction

Vagus nerve stimulation (VNS) is the most widely used non-pharmological treatment for drug-resistant epilepsy. Experiments in animal models of epilepsy and observations in human epilepsies demonstrate three temporal profiles of VNS antiseizure effects: (1) acute abortive effect, in which an ongoing seizure is attenuated by VNS applied during the seizure; (2) acute prophylactic effect, in which seizures are less likely to occur within minutes after a train of VNS than they would be in the absence of VNS, an effect that begins as soon as VNS is initiated; and (3) chronic progressive prophylactic effect, in which overall seizure frequency is reduced more after chronic VNS over weeks or months than occurred due to acute abortive and prophylactic effects. The mechanistic studies and clinical trials of VNS support regulatory approvals internationally, and provide greater information concerning VNS than is available for any other non-pharmological epilepsy therapy. The mechanistic investigations of VNS, which are the subject of this chapter, and the extensive clinical investigations and applications reviewed in subsequent chapters, justify consideration of VNS as a new epilepsy therapy.

A confluence of experimental and human data indicate that antiseizure actions of VNS are entirely based on alterations in brain function mediated through vagal afferents, with no participation of vagal visceroeffector activities. Vagal efferents underlie some of the common adverse effects of VNS, however. This chapter will first review the peripheral and central anatomy of the vagus and related systems, followed by considerations of experimental and clinical investigations of VNS mechanisms in the epilepsies.

Vagus nerve: course and composition

The vagus nerves carry somatic and visceral afferents and efferents. Most of the efferent fibers originate from neurons located in the medulla oblongata. Vagal efferents innervate striated muscles of the pharynx and larynx, and most of the thoracoabdominal viscera.[1,2] The two vagus nerves coalesce from multiple rootlets at the medulla, exit the skull in the jugular foramina, and traverse a long and winding route throughout the viscera. This complex and wide distribution earned the vagus nerve its name, as the Latin for 'wanderer.'

Each vagus nerve lies between the carotid artery and the jugular vein in the neck, within the carotid sheath (see Figure 1.1). In the cervical portion of the vagus nerve, unmyelinated, narrow-caliber C-fibers predominate over faster conducting, myelinated, intermediate-caliber B-fibers and thicker A-fibers.[3] Afferents compose about 80% of the fibers in the cervical portion of the vagus.[4] Most of the neurons that contribute afferent fibers to the cervical vagus have cell bodies located in two parasympathetic ganglia, the superior (jugular) vagal ganglion and the larger inferior (nodose) vagal ganglion, which are located at and immediately below the jugular foramen. A large population of special and general visceral afferents carry gustatory information, visceral sensory information, and other peripheral information. A limited number of vagal somatosensory afferents carry sensory information from skin on and near the ear.

Vagus nerve efferents

Most vagal efferents are parasympathetic projections to the heart, lungs, stomach and intestines, liver, pancreas, and kidneys. These efferents originate from preganglionic neurons of two pairs of nuclei in the medulla, the dorsal motor nucleus of the vagus and the nucleus ambiguus (see Figure 1.2). Vagal parasympathetic efferents synapse on neurons located in parasympathetic ganglia, which are located in or near the target organs. The vagus nerves are asymmetric with regards to cardiac innervation. The left vagus nerve carries most of the parasympathetic fibers that less densely innervate the ventricles, and the right vagus

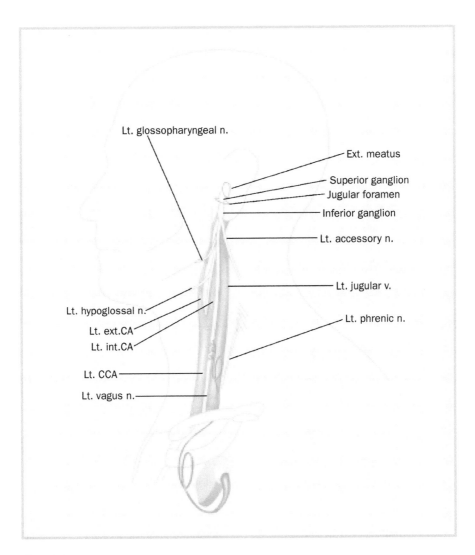

Figure 1.1
The cervical vagus nerve and vagus nerve stimulation. *Implantation site for contacts of the lead wire on the left vagus nerve is limited to the mid-inferior cervical region, as shown schematically. The nearby phrenic nerve might mistakenly be implanted instead of the left vagus, a rarely reported and poorly tolerated complication. Lt, Left; n., nerve; CCA, common carotid artery; CA, carotid artery; ext., external.*

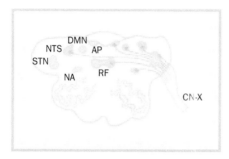

Figure 1.2
Schema of the dorsal medullary complex of the vagus. *The left vagus nerve's afferent fibers synapse on six nuclei of the dorsal medulla ipsilaterally, and also decussate to synapse on the contralateral nucleus of the tractus solitarius. Nerve terminations are indicated in blue, but most labels are placed on the homologous nucleus contralateral to the termination. NTS, Nucleus of the tractus solitarius; AP, area postrema; STN, spinal trigeminal nucleus; MRF, medullary reticular formation; DMN, dorsal motor nucleus of the vagus; NA, nucleus ambiguus.*

nerve carries most of the parasympathetic fibers that more densely innervate the cardiac atria.[5] Thus, vagal anatomy favors left (over right) vagus stimulation in order to avoid effects on cardiac rhythm. Actual measurements of cardiac rhythm with Holter monitoring, of respiratory function with pulmonary function tests, and of gastrointestinal parasympathetic effects with serum gastrin levels, show remarkably little vagal visceroeffector activity during therapeutic VNS in humans.[6–12] In one report, decreased myocardial contractility occurred in humans during intraoperative stimulation of distal branches of the vagus,[9] but stimulation

at this site appears to have limited relevance to cervical vagus stimulation. Cases of altered cardiac rhythm and altered respiration during cervical vagus stimulation have been reported to occur only during unusual states of intervention such as general anesthesia,[12] in patients with obstructive sleep apnea,[11] or in the absence of clinical manifestation.[10] As a group, these studies raise concern over possible adverse effects of VNS that may be specific to particular non-epileptic medical conditions involving viscera that receive vagal innervation. With the exception of obstructive sleep apnea, which has been the subject of one pilot study in patients receiving VNS,[11] VNS has not been studied in series of patients with cardiac arrhythmias, congestive heart failure, or other dysfunctions of vagally innervated organs.

Vagal branchiomotor efferents synapse as motor end plates on skeletal muscle fibers of the larynx and pharynx. The alpha-motoneurons of these efferent axons are located in the nucleus ambiguus of the medulla. Each vagus nerve contains efferents that innervate the vocal cord and other skeletal muscles of the larynx and pharynx unilaterally. Volitional swallowing does not appear to be affected by VNS using typical stimulation parameters, except for anecdotal reports of aspiration in children with severe cognitive and motor delay, when assisted feeding is performed during VNS. Vocalization is commonly altered by VNS, however. After upwards titration of current output, vocal stridor typically occurs during each train of stimulation.[6,13] VNS-induced vocal stridor is promptly reversible with a reduction in current density.

Afferent terminations and central pathways of the vagus nerve

Vagal afferent fibers enter the dorsolateral medulla and traverse the brainstem in the solitary tract. Most vagal afferents synapse in nuclei of the dorsal medullary complex of the vagus,[14–16] which includes the following structures of the medulla (see Figure 1.2):

- nucleus of the tractus solitarius (NTS);
- nucleus of the spinal tract of the trigeminal nerve;
- medial reticular formation of the medulla;
- area postrema;
- dorsal motor nucleus of the vagus;
- nucleus ambiguus.

The NTS receives the greatest number of vagal afferent synapses and each vagus nerve synapses bilaterally on the NTS. Each vagus nerve synapses only ipsilaterally in the other nuclei of the dorsal medullary complex of the vagus. The vagal afferents subserve visceral sensation (of the pharynx, larynx, trachea, and thoracoabdominal organs), somatic sensation (of a small patch of skin on and near the external ear), and taste (with receptors in the periepiglottal pharynx).

Vagal afferent synapses use the usual excitatory neurotransmitters (glutamate and aspartate) and inhibitory neurotransmitter (gamma-aminobutyric acid; GABA), and also use acetylcholine and a wide variety of neuropeptides.[17,18] As a group, these transmitters and modulators act very rapidly at neuronal membrane ion channels, and act more slowly via intraneuronal second messengers such as G-proteins.

NTS

The NTS extends as a tube-like structure above and below the vagal entry level, within the dorsal medulla and pons. In addition to dense innervation by the vagus nerves, the NTS also receives projections from a very wide range of peripheral and central sources.[1,2,15,19] These sources of afferents to the NTS include other peripheral nerves (the carotid sinus nerve, the aortic depressor nerve, and cranial nerves V, VII and IX), the spinal cord (via the spinosolitary tract), multiple brainstem structures (the area postrema, the rostral ventrolateral medulla, the parabrachial nucleus of the pons, the Kölliker-Fuse nucleus, the dorsal tegmental nucleus of the midbrain, and other sites), and cerebral structures (the paraventricular nucleus, lateral and posterior regions of the hypothalamus, and the central nucleus of the amygdala).

The NTS receives a wide range of somatic and visceral sensory information, receives projections from a diverse set of brainstem nuclei and cerebral structures, performs extensive information processing internally, projects to multiple hindbrain and forebrain structures, and produces motor and autonomic efferent outputs. For these reasons the NTS has been likened to a small brain within the larger brain. The vagus and associated sensory endings are the principal sensory organ of this small brain within a brain.

Vagal networks of the pons, midbrain, and cerebellum

Vagal afferents influence activities throughout a network of posterior fossa sites, with polysynaptic connections through the NTS and other nuclei. The NTS projects to a wide variety of structures within the posterior fossa,[1,2,20,21] as shown schematically in Figure 1.3, including all of the other nuclei of the dorsal medullary complex, the parabrachial nucleus and other pontine nuclei, the vermis and inferior portions of the cerebellar hemispheres, and the periaqueductal gray.

The NTS projects to the parabrachial nucleus of the pons most densely, and particular NTS subregions project specifically to different subnuclei of the parabrachial nucleus. Through disynaptic parabrachial relay projections, the NTS can influence

activities of respiratory pattern generation and pain modulation. Alterations in the respiratory pattern are not commonly observed during VNS, although patients with obstructive sleep apnea may in some cases experience increased apneas and hypopneas while asleep during high-frequency VNS.[11]

The periaqueductal gray is involved in central pain processing, and local alterations in processing during VNS may underlie antinociceptive effects of VNS in humans.[22] Through its own monosynaptic projections, the NTS can directly influence reflexes involving parasympathetic and sympathetic effector neurons, cranial nerve alpha-motoneurons, motor systems subserving posture and coordination, ascending visceral and somatic sensory pathways, and the local arousal system.

The area postrema also receives afferent synapses from the vagus nerve, from several other peripheral nerves, and from central autonomic structures.[1,2] The area postrema projects densely to the NTS and to the parabrachial nucleus, and less densely to the dorsal motor nucleus of the vagus, the nucleus ambiguus, and several other sites. The area postrema coordinates the vomiting reflex, and participates in cardiovascular, renovascular, and respiratory reflexes. The area postrema functions as an autonomic nucleus at the blood–brain interface, as one of the circumventricular organs.

Vagal afferents project to the

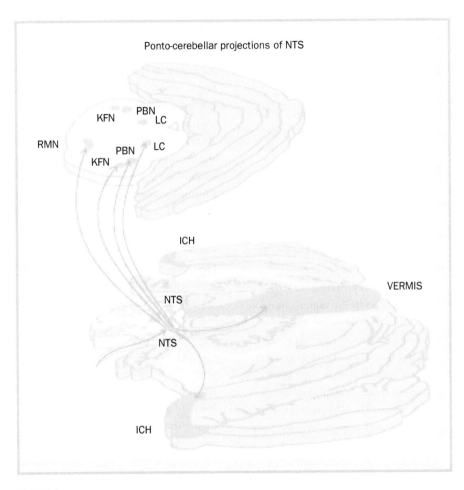

Figure 1.3
Schema of the bulbo–cerebellar polysynaptic projections of the nucleus of the tractus solitarius (NTS). *The left vagus nerve projects densely upon the NTS bilaterally, and the NTS projects to inferior and medial cerebellar regions, and to multiple pontine and mesencephalic nuclei. ICH, Inferior cerebellar hemisphere; KFN, Kölliker-Fuse nucleus; LC, locus coeruleus; RMN, raphe magnus nucleus; PBN, parabrachial nucleus.*

noradrenergic neuromodulatory systems of the brain and spinal cord via the NTS.[23] The locus coeruleus, a pontine nucleus, provides extremely widespread noradrenergic innervation of the entire cortex, diencephalon, and many other brain structures. The NTS projects to the locus coeruleus through two disynaptic pathways, an excitatory pathway via the nucleus paragigantocellularis and an inhibitory pathway via the nucleus prepositus hypoglossi.[24] Thus, VNS effects on the locus coeruleus might variably be excitatory, inhibitory or neutral.

Vagal afferents also project to the serotonergic neuromodulatory systems of the brain and spinal cord via the NTS.[23] Unlike the relatively compact locus coeruleus, the raphe nuclei are distributed amongst midline reticular neurons from the inferior medulla through the mesencephalon. The raphe nuclei provide extremely widespread serotonergic innervation of the entire cortex, diencephalon, and other brain structures. The NTS projects to multiple raphe nuclei, as do other nuclei of the dorsal medullary vagal complex, but the complexity of NTS–raphe pathways and transmitters is greater than for NTS–locus coeruleus interactions.[1,2] The locus coeruleus is the major source of norepinephrine and the raphe of serotonin in most of the brain. Vagal–locus coeruleus and vagal–raphe interactions are potentially relevant to VNS mechanisms, as norepinephrine, epinephrine, and serotonin exert antiseizure effects, among other actions.[25–28]

Vagal pathways in cerebral structures

A complex set of vagal pathways innervate limbic, reticular and autonomic centers of the cerebral hemispheres. The vagus nerve afferents have some disynaptic projections to the thalamus and hypothalamus via the NTS and the spinal trigeminal nucleus. Most of the widespread vagal projections to cerebral structures traverse three or more synapses (see Figures 1.4 and 1.5).

Vago–trigemino–thalamocortical processing mediates conscious laryngeal and pharyngeal sensation. Vagal sensory afferents synapse in the spinal trigeminal nucleus (STN), which projects unilaterally to somatosensory thalamic neurons of the contralateral ventral posteromedial (VPM) nucleus. These thalamic neurons project unilaterally to the inferior postcentral gyrus and inferior parietal lobule, which are ipsilateral to the VPM nucleus (and contralateral to the sensory receptors, and intermediary vagal sensory fibers and STN).[2] Predictably, increasing VNS output current can cause uncomfortable sensations, which are usually reported by the patient to be localized in the left throat, but occasionally are referred other sites in the left neck or left jaw. Uncomfortable sensations are rapidly reversible with current reduction.

The NTS projects to several structures within the cerebral hemispheres,[1,2] including

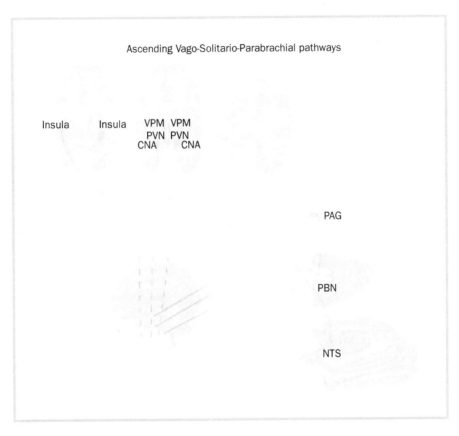

Figure 1.4
Schema of ascending bilateral vago–solitario–parabrachial pathways of the central autonomic, reticular activating and limbic systems. *Left vagal–bilateral nucleus of the tractus solitarius (NTS) projections, through synapses in the parabrachial nuclei, provide dense innervation of autonomic, reticular and limbic forebrain structures, as shown. Additional, more direct, NTS projections to the forebrain, and other polysynaptic pathways are discussed in the text. PBN, Parabrachial nucleus; PAG, periaqueductal gray; CNA, central nucleus of the amygdala; PVN, periventricular nucleus of the hypothalamus; VPM, ventral posteromedial nucleus of the thalamus.*

hypothalamic nuclei (the periventricular nucleus, the lateral hypothalamic area, and other nuclei), thalamic nuclei (including the

ventral posteromedial nucleus, paraventricular nucleus, and other nuclei), the central nucleus of the amygdala, the bed nucleus of the stria

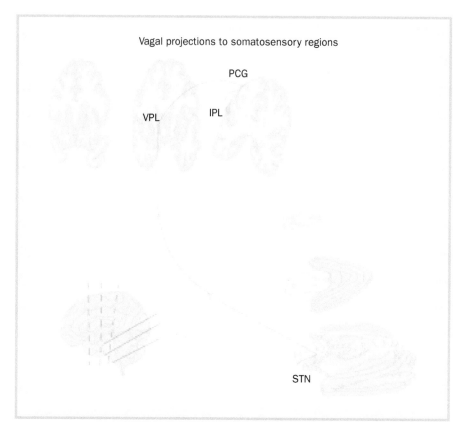

Figure 1.5
Schema of the ascending unilateral vago–trigemino–thalamocortical pathways of the somatosensory
system. Left vagal projections to the left spinal trigeminal nucleus subserve conscious sensation of deep
pharyngeal tissues and other modalities, as discussed in the text. STN, Spinal trigeminal nucleus; VPL,
ventral posterolateral nucleus of the thalamus; PCG, post-central gyrus; IPL, inferior parietal lobule.

terminalis, and the nucleus accumbens.
Through these projections, the NTS can
directly influence activities of extrapyramidal
motor systems, ascending visceral sensory

pathways, and higher autonomic systems.
Through its projection to the amygdala, the
NTS gains access to processes of the
amygdala–hippocampus–entorhinal cortex

loop of the limbic system, which are the sites that most often generate complex partial seizures.

The vagus–NTS–parabrachial pathways support additional higher cerebral influences of vagal afferents. The parabrachial nucleus projects to several structures within the cerebral hemispheres,[2,29] including the hypothalamus (particularly the lateral hypothalamic area), the thalamus (particularly intralaminar nuclei and the parvicellular portion of the ventral posteromedial nucleus), the amygdala (particularly the central nucleus of the amygdala, but also basolateral and other amygdalar nuclei), the anterior insula, and infralimbic cortex, lateral prefrontal cortex, and other cortical regions. The anterior insula constitutes the primary gustatory cortex. Higher order projections of the anterior insula are particularly dense in the inferior and inferolateral frontal cortices of the limbic system. The parabrachial nuclei function as major autonomic relay and processing sites for gustatory, pulmonary, and other autonomic information. Altered vagal sensory inputs to these systems may account for the occasional patient who experiences subjective dyspnea during VNS, which consistently occurs in the absence of objective changes in pulmonary function.[7]

The medial reticular formation of the medulla receives afferent projections from the vagus nerve and from many other sources. The medial reticular formation of the medulla projects to the nucleus reticularis thalami (a thalamic nucleus that projects to most of the other thalamic nuclei and exerts strong influences on synchronization of thalamocortical projections) and to the intralaminar nuclei of the thalamus (the centromedian and other thalamic nuclei that have extremely widespread projections to the cerebral cortex and the striatum).[1,2,29,30] The thalamic reticular formation serves to coordinate many cortical activities [including generation of sleep spindles and slow electroencephalogram (EEG) waves of sleep via diffuse thalamocortical projections] through diffuse projections to cerebral structures, but also has strong influences throughout the brainstem via descending projections.[31–33] Patients often report improved alertness during VNS. A study of epilepsy patients, who did not have sleep disorders, revealed improved diurnal alertness during VNS; improved alertness was independent of seizure reductions.[34] Improved reticular activating system function must mediate improved alertness, although the mechanisms of VNS alterations in arousal are unclear.

Hypothesis of seizure antagonism by vagus nerve stimulation (VNS)

In 1985, Zabara[35] first proposed that cervical VNS might attenuate seizures by desynchronizing electrocerebral activities. Early neurophysiological studies had shown that cervical VNS can induce EEG desynchronization in cats.[36] Cortical and thalamocortical neuronal interactions become abnormally hypersynchronized during seizures in animal models of partial and generalized epilepsies.[37,38] Intracerebral recordings in humans, performed for presurgical evaluation of medically refractory partial epilepsies, demonstrate hypersynchrony among multiple cortical sites during seizures.[39] Zabara[35] postulated that desynchronizing these overly synchronized activities would confer antiseizure effects on VNS. Empirical observations in animal models of epilepsy subsequently demonstrated antiseizure effects of VNS. Preclinical safety studies of VNS examined general effects of cervical VNS on brain function in animals.

Experimental studies of vagus nerve stimulation (VNS)

General effects of VNS on brain function

Localized alterations in neuronal function may or may not occur at a particular site that is connected with the vagus nerve by polysynaptic pathways in response to electrical stimulation of the cervical vagus nerve. Additional investigation is required to determine whether VNS actually affects sites that are anatomically accessible to vagal

influences. Naritoku et al[40] showed that cervical VNS, with stimulation parameters as used in therapeutic VNS, can in fact alter multiregional neuronal activities of the brainstem and cortex. They measured neuronal *fos* expression to determine overall neuronal biochemical activity in healthy rats (which were not caused to have seizures). The rats received VNS for 3 hours before sacrifice and immunomapping of *fos*, a neuronal nuclear protein that has increased concentrations at sites of increased overall biochemical activity. Control groups either did not receive any electrical stimulation or received electrical stimulation of tissues near but not in the vagus nerve. Intermittent VNS caused acute increases in neuronal *fos* expression in the medullary vagal complex, the locus coeruleus, several thalamic and hypothalamic nuclei, the amygdala, and cingulate and retrosplenial cortex, on comparison with the control group *fos* distributions.[40]

Function of the reticular activating system, in generating wake–sleep states and other aspects of thalamocortical interaction, can be studied with extracranial or intracranial EEG recordings. As previously noted, under general anesthesia cats demonstrated EEG desynchronization during VNS in the earliest reported experiment.[36] Later studies showed that VNS can also induce increased EEG synchronization in non-epileptic animals, depending on the frequency of stimulation.[41–43] These studies also showed that VNS reduced or abolished interictal epileptiform activities that were induced by focal cortical application of strychnine[43] or penicillin[42] in the absence of induced seizures.

The remarkable paucity of peripheral parasympathetic effects of therapeutic VNS has been addressed in experimental studies. The apparent basis of preferential activation of afferents over efferents during therapeutic VNS may be partly due to the quantitative predominance of afferent over efferent fibers in the cervical portion of the vagus, as discussed above, but it also is clear that therapeutic VNS does not much affect the unmyelinated vagal parasympathetic efferent fibers. The vagus nerves contain A-, B- and C-fibers, as histopathologically defined by diameter and myelination.[3,44] The vagal A-fibers (the largest and most heavily myelinated fibers) have the lowest amplitude-duration threshold required for VNS to excite action potentials, with higher thresholds for B-fiber excitation, and highest thresholds to excite the narrow, unmyelinated C-fibers.[44] These studies also showed that, in anesthetized rats, effects on heart rate (bradycardia) and respiration (apnea or hypopnea) occurred only at VNS thresholds sufficient to excite action potentials in C-fibers.[44] The nearly complete absence of parasympathetic visceral effects during human VNS and other indirect evidence are concordant with the principle that C-fibers are not excited or are minimally excited during therapeutic VNS.

Chemically induced tremors were suppressed during left cervical VNS in the rodent harmaline tremor model.[45] The mechanism by which VNS might suppress tremor remains unclear.

Behavioral effects of VNS have not been fully studied in animals (or in humans). An interesting pair of rodent and human studies by Clark et al[46,47] showed evidence of improved learning and memory during clinically relevant levels of VNS. A footshock avoidance task was learned by rats implanted with vagus nerve electrodes, and immediately after training rats received either VNS or sham stimulation. The rats that received VNS retained the task performance after 24 hours significantly better than did the control group. Performance improvements were associated more with intermediate than with highest or lowest amplitudes of VNS in these studies.[47]

Experimental VNS studies of antiseizure effects

Three temporal patterns of seizure antagonism are observed in animal studies of VNS:

- **acute abortive effect**, in which an ongoing seizure is attenuated by VNS applied after seizure onset;
- **acute prophylactic effect**, in which seizure-inducing insults are less effective in provoking seizures when applied within minutes after the end of a train of VNS

than these insults would be in the absence of VNS, or at longer periods after VNS;

• **chronic progressive prophylactic effect**, in which total seizure counts (totaled continuously over long periods between and during intermittent VNS) are reduced more after chronic stimulation over weeks or months than after acute stimulation over < 1 day.

Animal studies also show that VNS can antagonize the development of epilepsy in the kindling model of epileptogenesis.

Acute abortive antiseizure effects of VNS were established in several experimental models of acute symptomatic seizures in rats, dogs and monkeys. These studies used maximal electroshocks to the head, and the systemic proconvulsants pentylenetetrazol and strychnine, to induce seizures.[42,44,48,49] These are the same acute insults most often used to screen potential AEDs for antiseizure efficacy. These studies consistently showed that after a seizure began, it could be stopped or attenuated with application of VNS during the seizure. Presumably the mechanisms of acute abortive effects in animals underlie the seizure-attenuating effects of external magnetic (non-automated) stimulation, in which some patients reportedly can prevent a complex partial seizure when VNS is activated during an aura, or can have an observer prevent secondary generalization when VNS is activated during a complex partial seizure.

Acute prophylactic antiseizure effects of VNS also were established in acute epilepsy models, which demonstrated that antiseizure effects of VNS outlast the period of nerve stimulation. Takaya et al[48] examined the temporal profile of post-stimulation seizure antagonism in detail. In rats with seizures induced by pentylenetetrazol, which was administered at various intervals after the end of a train of VNS, they found anticonvulsant effects that declined gradually over 10 minutes after VNS. They also suggested the possibility of a chronic prophylactic effect, in that greater anticonvulsant effects occurred after longer, cumulative periods of intermittent VNS, even within the short durations of study in this acute epilepsy model. Together, the acute experiments showed that antiseizure effects of VNS were greater at frequencies of stimulation > 10 Hz and < 60 Hz for both acute abortive and acute prophylactic effects. Presumably the mechanisms of acute prophylactic effects in animals underlie the main seizure-attenuating effects of automated stimulation, in which patients receive trains of VNS at regular intervals without gating of stimulation to seizure occurrence, but nonetheless begin to experience reduction of seizures as soon as VNS begins.

Chronic prophylactic antiseizure effects of VNS were established in a chronic primate epilepsy model, which found that antiseizure effects of VNS continued to increase after weeks of VNS. In this chronic model of neocortical epilepsy, VNS abolished or reduced seizures due to topical instillation of cobalt on the neocortex in primates.[50] Unlike VNS in subprimate models of epilepsy, this study did not find that VNS reduced interictal spikes, despite antiseizure effects in these monkeys.[50] These primate studies showed both acute and chronic prophylactic effects of VNS. Presumably the mechanisms of chronic progressive prophylactic effects in monkeys also underlie the main seizure-attenuating effects of automated stimulation, in that many patients experience incremental reduction of seizures over many months after VNS begins.

Antiepileptogenic effects of VNS were established in a recent study of VNS in amygdala kindling. Pretreatment with VNS markedly reduced amygdala kindling in cats, demonstrating the ability of VNS to antagonize the development of epilepsy during ongoing brain insult in this chronic model of temporal lobe epilepsy.[51] Presumably antiepileptogenic effects might also occur in humans, but there are no reports of VNS applied before the first seizure in humans who subsequently receive potentially epileptogenic insults, nor is it possible to readily evaluate ongoing epileptogenesis in patients who already have established epilepsy. Thus, the possibility of antiepileptogenic effects in humans remains theoretical.

Experimental VNS studies of antiseizure mechanisms

Peripheral, efferent vagal parasympathetic effects do not mediate antiseizure actions of VNS, based on two critical mechanistic experiments. Zabara[49] found that acute antiseizure VNS effects were not reversed by transection of the vagus nerve distally to the cervical site of vagal stimulation in dogs with motor seizures induced by systemic strychnine or pentylenetetrazol. Krahl et al[52] chemically lesioned the vagal efferents just distal to the site of cervical stimulation in rats. This study was based on the observation that essentially all vagal efferents below the cervical stimulation site are C-fibers. Capsaicin was used to chemically destroy the C-fibers without affecting larger myelinated (afferent) vagal fibers. Systemic pentylenetetrazol induced seizures in lesion and control groups, and then VNS was used to attenuate the pentylenetetrazol-induced seizure. VNS attenuated seizures equally well, whether or not vagal C-fibers had been destroyed.[52]

The brainstem and cerebral pathways of polysynaptic vagal projections must be individually investigated to elucidate VNS mechanisms. The role of the NTS in regulating epileptic excitability was investigated in a recent study.[53] Various manipulations of GABA and glutamate neurotransmission within the NTS, each with the effect of inhibiting NTS output, were shown to reduce susceptibility of rats to seizure induction by systemic pentylenetetrazol, by systemic bicuculline, and by focal infusion of bicuculline into the area tempestas. Based on this functional study and the extensive investigations of vagal afferent pathways, it seems clear the NTS must transmit and modulate VNS antiseizure actions. Further studies of NTS function during VNS and control states of epilepsy models will be necessary.

The locus coeruleus was shown to mediate acute VNS antiseizure effects in an investigation using the rodent maximal electroshock model.[54] Acute antiseizure effects of VNS were similar to those of other studies in the control groups of this study. The antiseizure effects of VNS were fully reversed by infusion of lidocaine into the locus coeruleus bilaterally. Since lidocaine might diffuse away from the site of injection, and anesthetize nearby fiber tracts or nuclei of the pons, the investigators then created a chemical lesion highly specific to noradrenergic neurons. After chronically depleting norepinephrine in the locus coeruleus, by infusing 6-hydroxydopamine into the locus coeruleus bilaterally, the acute VNS antiseizure effects again were fully reversed.[54] Similar lesion studies of other sites in the vagal projection pathways have not been reported, nor have mechanistic studies using chronic experimental models that are more similar to human epilepsies. Nonetheless, the locus

coeruleus and noradrenergic actions must be primary targets of future mechanistic studies of VNS.

Electrophysiological studies of vagus nerve stimulation (VNS) in humans

Electroencephalography

Four publications have reported effects of VNS on the human EEG. Nine partial epilepsy patients at the University of Florida had scalp EEG recordings before and after chronic VNS, with comparison of EEG both by visual interpretation and quantitative frequency analysis.[55] Normal EEG activities were unchanged during VNS, and were also unchanged during non-stimulation periods after chronic VNS when compared with pre-VNS baseline EEG. Interictal epileptiform EEG activities were unchanged from baseline during VNS and during non-stimulation periods after chronic VNS, both in patients with very frequent spikes and in those with only occasional spikes. Electrographic seizures abruptly ceased during a train of VNS in two patients who were able to abort behavioral seizures when the stimulator was activated manually during auras.

In another study, six partial epilepsy patients had scalp EEG recordings during maximal arousal, before VNS began and following > 6 months of chronic VNS.[56] Series of EEG acquisitions consisted of three epochs lasting 60 seconds each, recorded sequentially just before a train of VNS, during VNS and just after VNS. Visual interpretation of the EEG under the baseline, activation, and post-activation conditions did not show any changes across these conditions in any individual. Quantitative frequency analysis of activities at each of the standard 10–20 system electrodes did not show significant differences in total power across these conditions in any individual. Even with averaging of quantified data across the entire group, no significant differences by condition were shown for total power, median frequency, or power in any of the standard frequency bands. These two studies used different methods, but neither study found evidence of EEG desynchronization during VNS, or of significant quantitative effects of VNS on the human EEG.

A case report of a patient undergoing presurgical evaluation with intrahippocampal electrodes noted apparent effects of VNS on baseline frequency of interictal epileptiform discharges.[57] Baseline rates of hippocampal spiking decreased during VNS at 30 Hz, but increased during VNS at 5 Hz.

Reductions in interictal epileptiform activity during chronic VNS also were reported by Koo.[58] She studied a population with quite different characteristics from those of the two earlier series. Unlike patients in the earlier scalp EEG studies, her patients had

both generalized-onset and partial-onset seizures, had greater frequencies of interictal discharges at baseline, and were younger. In this report, both generalized and focal spikes were diminished during 12 months of VNS therapy. Spikes were manually counted, without computerized spike detection or automated analyses of background scalp EEG activities. Spike reduction did not correlate well with seizure reduction. Thus, this study provided indirect evidence of VNS interference with hypersynchronous, thalamocortically mediated spike generation, but did not show definite relevance of this action to seizure reduction.

Scalp EEG potentials evoked by VNS

Cervical VNS can be investigated by recording cerebral evoked potentials (EPs), using scalp EEG recording and stimulus-gated averaging techniques similar to those used to measure visual, auditory and somatosensory EPs.[59,60] Hammond et al[59] recorded a single surface-negative potential of high amplitude, which had a peak at about 12 milliseconds from onset of VNS and had a very widespread field. Topographic mapping over craniocervical regions revealed that the VNS EPs had a maximum over the left cervical region. The electrical generators of the scalp potentials were subsequently shown to be left anterior cervical skeletal muscles. The VNS EPs were abolished on administration of a neuromuscular blocking agent, and VNS EPs returned after effects of neuromuscular blockade were reversed. Thus, no VNS EPs of cerebral origin were recorded when using VNS parameters similar to those used for epilepsy therapy.

Stimulation of the left cervical vagus nerve at higher amplitudes (up to 14 mA) than those used in epilepsy therapy can be used to elicit VNS EPs of cerebral origin.[60] A series of three surface-negative potentials at about 71, 194, and 328 milliseconds from stimulus onset were recorded using scalp electrodes. Similar results were obtained on electrical stimulation of the esophagus, with slightly longer latencies to all three surface-negative peaks in epileptic than in healthy subjects. The differing latencies between epileptic and healthy subjects were attributed by the investigators to effects of AED in slowing neural conduction.

Effects of VNS on visual, auditory, and somatosensory EPs

The effects of acute and chronic VNS on other EPs have also been studied.[59,61] In nine patients, Hammond et al[59] found no effects of acute or chronic VNS on visual, somatosensory, brainstem auditory, 40-Hz auditory, or P300 auditory ('cognitive') EPs. In three patients, Naritoku et al[61] found no effects of chronic VNS on brainstem auditory EPs, but did find prolongation of the latency from the N13 to N20 peaks (often considered to represent central projections to thalamocortical areas) of median nerve somatosensory EPs. Both groups used similar techniques to record median nerve somatosensory EPs, so it is difficult to explain their divergent results.

Cerebral blood flow (CBF) studies of vagus nerve stimulation (VNS) in humans

Non-invasive mapping of anatomical sites of increased or decreased synaptic activity can be performed with functional imaging of CBF. Rapidly occurring changes in regional CBF mainly reflect changes in transsynaptic neurotransmission in the absence of seizures, cerebral vasospasm, arterial thromboembolism, and other brain vascular dysfunctions.[62] Regional CBF maps can be constructed from data acquired with positron emission tomography (PET), single photon emission computed tomography (SPECT) or functional magnetic resonance imaging (fMRI). Temporal and spatial resolutions, and many other characteristics, differ among PET, SPECT and fMRI data. The CBF measurements made with SPECT reflect a duration of CBF that is longer than one train of therapeutic VNS, so SPECT either determines CBF during combined stimulation and post-stimulation periods, or determines CBF during interstimulation periods only.

Both PET and fMRI can resolve CBF during time periods as brief as one typical train of therapeutic VNS, and fMRI can resolve CBF during time periods as short as a single pulse of therapeutic VNS. The timing of onset and offset of one train of VNS can be correlated with adequate precision to CBF data acquisition with PET in order to permit CBF measurements during stimulation without including periods between trains of stimulation. The MRI environment and the characteristics of current VNS stimulation systems do not permit triggering of single pulses of VNS to magnetic signal pulse acquisitions, and it is difficult to record VNS pulses electrically in the MRI environment in order to permit precise temporal correlation of VNS pulse onset with MRI signals. However, patient perception of onset of a train of VNS pulses can be used to time MRI during stimulation without including periods between stimulation. While SPECT does not permit intrasubject statistical testing of differences between repeated CBF measures during a single session in one subject, this can be achieved with PET or with fMRI.

Altered synaptic activities during VNS have most often been studied with PET. Activation PET methods were validated theoretically and technically in numerous PET studies comparing regional distributions of $[^{15}O]H_2O$ with and without particular motor and cognitive tasks, and sensory stimuli.[63–67] For example, PET studies showed unilateral thalamic, postcentral gyral and opercular CBF increases during focal somatosensory stimulation, with CBF increases contralateral to the side of somatic sensory stimulation.[64–66] Visceral sensory activation PET studies found increased $[^{15}O]H_2O$ activity bilaterally in the thalami, and the pre- and post-central gyri, during intrarectal balloon dilation.[68] Thus, PET imaging of CBF during VNS can be used to look for brain regions that significantly change levels of information processing during VNS.

Changes in CBF induced by acute VNS

Acute effects of VNS on regional synaptic activities were investigated at Emory University by comparing repeated measurements of baseline CBF (without stimulation) and repeated measurements of CBF during trains of stimulation, with intra- and intersubject statistical analysis of PET data (see Figure 1.6).[69] In these studies the stimulation onset was gated to the time of arrival of $[^{15}O]H_2O$ in cerebral arteries following intravenous bolus administration of the radioligand, and emission scan acquisition was gated to the time of actual stimulation. Acute VNS activation PET studies used baseline scans that were performed just before VNS was started for the first time (at 2 weeks following device implantation) and scans recorded during trains of VNS, within 20

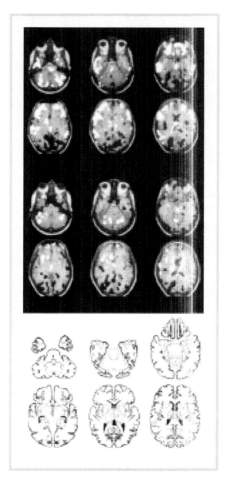

Figure 1.6
Activation [^{15}O]H$_2$O PET studies of acute vagus nerve stimulation (VNS). *Data were obtained first with the stimulator shut off, then during VNS, within the first day after chronic VNS began (using techniques described by Henry et al[69]). Volumes of blood flow increases (in yellow) and decreases (in blue), which have T-values ≥5, are superimposed on gray-scale MRI scans. The subjects' left is displayed on the right-hand image. The first two rows consist of axial images with approximately 1 cm spacing, arranged from inferior (upper left) to superior (lower right), of the high-stimulation group (n = 5). The middle two rows are similarly arranged data for the low-stimulation group (n = 5). The bottom two rows are axial brain schemata at the same levels as for the other rows, with numbers inserted to indicate the locations of these structures: 1, dorsal–rostral medulla; 2/3, left/right inferior cerebellar hemisphere; 4, cerebellar vermis; 5, hypothalamus; 6/7, left/right thalamus; 8/9, left/right hippocampus; 10/11, left/right amygdala; 12/13, left/right cingulate gyrus; 14/15, left/right insula; 16/17, left/right orbitofrontal cortex; 18/19, left/right inferior frontal gyrus; 20/21, left/right entorhinal cortex; 22/23, left/right temporal pole; 24/25, left/right inferior postcentral gyrus; 26/27, left/right inferior parietal lobule. (Figure used with permission from Henry et al.[69])*

hours after VNS was initiated.[69] Parameters for VNS were at high levels for five patients and low levels for five patients. Statistical testing analyzed the differences between the baseline scans and the VNS activation scans, both within individuals and also in groups of patients. Significant blood flow increases in the dorsal–central–rostral medulla, which is the site of the dorsal medullary vagal complex (the NTS and five other nuclei that receive vagal afferent terminations), were induced by VNS, in both the high- and low-stimulation groups.

In these studies the high-stimulation group had larger regions of activation (increased CBF during VNS) and deactivation (decreased CBF during VNS, compared with baseline CBF) over both cerebral hemispheres than did the low-stimulation group.[69] In both groups, regional blood flow changes during acute VNS demonstrated sites of increased synaptic activity in the right thalamus and right postcentral gyrus (the 'sensory strip'), which are the major sites of cerebral processing of left-sided somatic sensation. This is not surprising, since all of the patients reported feeling the left cervical tingling sensations that normally occur during VNS. Most of the cortical and subcortical regions that had altered blood flow during VNS are not involved in sensory processing, however. Both high- and low-stimulation groups had VNS-activated sites in the inferior cerebellar hemispheres bilaterally.

Multiple cerebral structures had altered CBF during acute VNS, and affected structures were those most densely innervated by polysynaptic vagal pathways in reticular, autonomic and limbic systems. Significant blood flow increases occurred in the hypothalami, and left and right anterior insular cortices in both groups. The high-stimulation group had significant blood flow increases in the left and right orbitofrontal gyri, right entorhinal cortex and the right temporal pole, which did not occur in the low-stimulation group. Both groups had significant decreases in amygdalar, hippocampal and posterior cingulate gyral blood flow, which were bilateral in each case. It is of some interest that the amygdala and hippocampus had bilaterally reduced synaptic activity during VNS, since these regions are often involved early on in complex partial seizures. It can be postulated that regions of VNS-induced synaptic activity decreases might have a lower probability of sustaining repetitive ictal firing, due to decreased excitatory synaptic activity.

Thalamic activations occurred bilaterally in both high- and low-stimulation groups during VNS. Numerous thalamic nuclei contain thalamocortical relay neurons, which as a group project to all cortical areas and essentially all subcortical structures.[32] Normal activities of 'specific' thalamocortical relay neurons transmit pre-processed sensory information to higher levels and pre-processed motor commands to lower levels. Both 'specific' and 'non-specific' thalamocortical relay neurons drive the entire cortex through the various waking and sleep states, and synchronize cortical electrical rhythms, among many other thalamic processes that initiate or modulate cortical activities.[33,39] It was postulated that VNS might cause the thalamic activities that prevent seizure onset, or that terminate or limit propagation of electrocortical seizure activities.

Bilateral thalamic CBF increases during acute VNS are strongly correlated with the individual's responsiveness to chronic VNS.[70] Among 11 patients who had acute VNS activation PET studies, individuals showed improvements in seizure frequency over a wide range, with as much as 71% seizure reduction during 3 months of chronic VNS. Patients' AEDs were not increased during the 3 months of chronic VNS. Intrasubject comparisons of CBF during acute VNS and baseline CBF were performed with T-statistical mapping. Changes in frequency of complex partial seizures (with or without secondary generalization) and T-threshold regional CBF changes (for each of the 25 regions of previously observed significant CBF change) were rank ordered across patients. Spearman rank correlation coefficients measured associations of seizure-frequency change and T-threshold regional CBF change. Many cerebral regions had significant changes in CBF during VNS, but only the right and left thalami showed significant associations of CBF change with seizure responsiveness. Increased CBF in the thalami correlated with decreased seizures ($P < 0.001$). These findings support the concept that therapeutic VNS antagonizes seizures by actions that increase synaptic activities in the thalami bilaterally.

The immediate post-stimulation effects of acute VNS on regional CBF were studied by Vonck et al[71] using SPECT. These

investigators used paired ^{99m}Tc-ethyl cysteinate dimer and SPECT scans in each subject, with one scan at baseline before VNS began and the other within 1 hour later, with radioligand injection just at the end of the first train of VNS. This SPECT study found significantly decreased left thalamic and left parietal CBF on VNS-activated scans. The VNS current intensity averaged less in the SPECT study than in the earlier PET studies, and the PET studies had a longer period of VNS (intermittently over < 1 day) before the VNS-activated scans were obtained. The PET and SPECT imaging techniques are themselves quite different, which may account for the divergent results. Nonetheless, taken together, the PET and SPECT data suggest that during VNS the thalami and other regions have increased CBF, and immediately after VNS these regions have decreased CBF, compared with baseline.

fMRI can be used to study the time course of regional CBF alteration during VNS in detail, as reported in depressed patients who do not have seizures.[72] These studies are technically challenging, but feasibility in epilepsy was shown in a study of four patients.[73] This study found multiple cortical regions of increased blood flow during VNS in each patient, but blood flow increases were inconsistently found in the thalami and other subcortical regions. The temporal resolution of fMRI might permit analysis of the time course of local blood flow changes after single pulses of VNS, if gating of MRI signal analysis to VNS pulse onset and offset can be achieved with future technical developments.

Changes in CBF induced by chronic VNS

Chronic effects of VNS on regional CBF have been studied in patients after months or years of intermittent VNS.[74–76] Garnett et al[74] averaged PET data of five patients, and found increased blood flow in the left thalamus and left anterior cingulate gyrus during chronic VNS. Two of their five patients had seizures during image acquisition. Complex, multiregional alterations in CBF occur during and shortly after complex partial seizures,[77] which makes interpretation of these PET results difficult. Ko et al[76] averaged PET data of three patients and found that chronic VNS increased blood flow in the right thalamus, the right posterior temporal cortex, the left putamen, and the left inferior cerebellum. Their findings may have been influenced by prior epilepsy surgery, with right anterior temporal lobectomy in one case and left frontal resection in another.

The Emory group performed chronic VNS activation PET studies on the same 10 patients who had acute VNS activation PET, as reviewed above. After 3 months of chronic, intermittent VNS, each patient again had three control scans without VNS and three scans during 30 seconds of VNS.[75] Data were analyzed in the same fashion as for the acute VNS activation studies. In general, the high- and low-stimulation groups both had smaller volumes of significant activations during the chronic studies than they did during the acute studies. During acute and chronic studies, VNS-induced CBF increases had the same distributions over the right postcentral gyrus, and bilateral thalami, hypothalami, inferior cerebellar hemispheres, and inferior parietal lobules. During acute studies, VNS decreased bilateral hippocampal, amygdalar and cingulate CBF, and increased bilateral insular CBF; these regions had no significant VNS-induced CBF changes during the chronic study; (the mean seizure frequency decrease was 38% between the acute and chronic PET studies.) Thus, seizure control improved during a period over which some acute VNS-induced CBF changes declined (mainly over cortical regions), while other VNS-induced CBF changes persisted (mainly over subcortical regions).

Differences between acute and chronic VNS activation PET studies may reflect brain adaptation to chronic stimulation of the left vagus nerve. Therapeutic VNS often causes gradually improving seizure control over periods > 3 months (and, in some cases, over periods > 1 year), even when VNS parameters are not modified over the period of improvement in seizure frequency.[78,79] Further study will be required to determine why acute effects of VNS on brain blood flow differ from VNS effects after months or years of stimulation. Intrasubject differences between acute and chronic VNS activation scans may reveal processes of adaptation to chronic VNS. Correlation of acute-to-chronic adaptation of regional CBF during VNS with chronic changes in seizure frequency, may suggest that some of these processes have an antiepileptic effect. Ultimately, animal experiments will be necessary to elucidate the mechanisms of any such effects.

Cerebrospinal fluid studies of vagus nerve stimulation (VNS) in humans

Chronic VNS is associated with alterations in cerebrospinal fluid (CSF) amino acid and phospholipid content.[80,81] The latter of these studies had a larger patient group and longer follow-up of antiseizure efficacy. Ben-Menachem et al[81] examined CSF chemistry before and after 3 months of therapeutic VNS, in groups receiving high versus low stimulation levels, and studied the same groups again 6 months later, after all 16 subjects received high levels of VNS. Subjects were stratified by levels of stimulation and by responsiveness of their seizures to VNS therapy. Overall, CSF concentrations of total and free GABA increased significantly in all patients at 3 months, with greater increases in the group with lower stimulation at 3 months and greater increases in the non-responders at

9 months. The entire patient group had decreased CSF concentrations of the excitatory amino acids glutamate and aspartate at 9 months, and increased CSF concentrations of the serotonin metabolite 5-hydroxyindoleacetic acid (5-HIAA), but these changes did not reach statistical significance at 3 or 9 months. The relationship of these findings to the mechanism of VNS antiepileptic action is uncertain, owing in part to the fact that non-responders had greater excitatory amino acid decreases, and non-responders had greater GABA and 5-HIAA increases, than did the subjects whose seizures responded most to chronic VNS. Thus, while these changes in CSF amino acids is probably actioned by chronic VNS on neurotransmitter release, it is not clear that these actions are antiepileptic. On the other hand, significant CSF increases in the cell membrane phospholipid precursor ethanolamine were greatest in the high-stimulation group at 3 months, and in the responders at 3 and 9 months. The authors suggest that increased CSF ethanolamine levels may be a sign of increased turnover of neuronal membrane components.[81] Currently it is unclear how increased neuronal membrane synthesis might relate to improved seizure control.

Putative mechanisms of antiepileptic drugs (AED) and vagus nerve stimulation (VNS) in human epilepsies

The desired antiseizure actions of VNS may be mediated: (1) through increased synaptic activities in the thalamus and thalamocortical projection pathways bilaterally, leading to increased arousal and possibly to decreased synchrony of synaptic activities between and within cortical regions; (2) through intermittently increased synaptic activities in the insula, hypothalamus, and other components of the central autonomic system; (3) through transiently decreased synaptic activities in the amygdala, hippocampus, and other components of the limbic system; and (4) through intermittently increased release of norepinephrine (and perhaps also of serotonin) over widespread cerebral regions. In contrast, the major antiseizure actions of AEDs include: (1) limitation of the maximal ictal rates of sustained repetitive firing of neuronal action potentials, by decreasing conductance at voltage-sensitive sodium ionophores; (2) inhibitory hyperpolarization of postsynaptic neuronal membranes, by prolonging the duration of openings or increasing the frequency of openings of the chloride ionophores that are linked with $GABA_A$ receptors so as to increase overall chloride conductance; and (3) reduction of hypersynchronous cortical spike-wave

discharges, by reducing low-threshold (T-type) calcium currents of thalamocortical relay neurons.[82] It is unlikely that VNS would reduce cortical hypersynchrony by direct effects on calcium channel conductance in membranes of thalamocortical relay neurons, similar to effects of ethosuximide and other anti-absence agents. It is likely that altered polysynaptic activities of the vago–solitario–parabrachial pathways mediate altered activities of thalamocortical relay neurons during VNS, and that anti-absence agents do not have such actions. While some AEDs may exert adrenergic agonism, it is not clear that any AEDs use adrenergic agonism as the predominant antiseizure action. Thus, the antiseizure effects of VNS and AEDs appear to be largely distinct.

The mechanisms of toxicity and adverse effects also differ significantly between VNS and commonly used AEDs, as do the empirically observed occurrences of adverse effects. For example, sedative effects and impaired cognition are commonly observed with the use of AEDs that increase GABAergic inhibition or that reduce rapid, repeated interneuronal action potentials by limiting sodium conductance; these adverse effects are rarely, if ever, attributable to VNS. Voice changes often occur during activation of vagal efferents to the left vocal cord by VNS, but not by AEDs effects. Further, complex pharmacokinetic interactions among AEDs and other pharmacological agents appear entirely unaffected by VNS. Current understandings of therapeutic mechanisms strongly support the common-sense interpretation of the clinical studies: adjunctive VNS can add antiseizure effect to any AED regimen, with no interactive toxicity, and no effect on drug distribution and elimination.

Summary and conclusions

No single mechanism of action has been shown to mediate antiseizure effects of VNS. Anatomical pathways provide the left cervical vagus afferent and efferent fibers with access to: (1) parasympathetic control of the heart and multiple other visceral organs; (2) pharyngeal muscles of vocalization; (3) a limited somatosensory representation of the head and neck; and (4) a widespread array of autonomic, reticular and limbic structures of the brainstem and both hemispheres. Therapeutic VNS appears to have remarkably little affect on the vagal parasympathetic visceroeffectors. The common, reversible, adverse effects of VNS mainly involve vocalization and somatic sensation. Experimental and human studies most strongly support altered activities of the reticular activating system, the central autonomic network, the limbic system, and the diffuse noradrenergic projection system as modalities of seizure antagonism.

References

1. Nieuwenhuys R, Voogd J, van Huijzen C. The Human Central Nervous System, 3rd edn (Springer-Verlag: Berlin, 1988.)

2. Parent A. Carpenter's Human Neuroanatomy, 9th edn (Williams & Wilkins: Baltimore, 1996.)

3. Agostini E, Chinnock JE, Daly MS, Murray JG. Functional and histological studies of the vagus nerve and its branches to the heart, lungs, and abdominal viscera in the cat. J Physiol 1957; 135:182–205.

4. Foley JO, DuBois F. Quantitative studies of the vagus nerve in the cat. I. The ratio of sensory and motor fibers. J Comp Neurol 1937; 67:49–97.

5. Saper CB, Kibbe MR, Hurley KM et al. Brain natriuretic peptide-like immunoreactive innervation of the cardiovascular and cerebrovascular systems in the rat. Circ Res 1990; 67:1345–54.

6. Handforth A, DeGiorgio CM, Schachter SC et al. Vagus nerve stimulation therapy for partial-onset seizures: a randomized, active-control trial. Neurology 1998; 51:48–55.

7. Banzett RB, Guz A, Paydarfar D et al. Cardiorespiratory variables and sensation during stimulation of the left vagus in patients with epilepsy. Epilepsy Res 1999; 35:1–11.

8. Binks AP, Paydarfar D, Schachter SC et al. High strength stimulation of the vagus nerve in awake humans: a lack of cardiorespiratory effects. Respir Physiol 2001; 127:125–33.

9. Lewis ME, Al-Khalidi AH, Bonser RS et al. Vagus nerve stimulation decreases left ventricular contractility in vivo in the human and pig heart. J Physiol 2001; 534:547–52.

10. Frei MG, Osorio I. Left vagus nerve

stimulation with the neurocybernetic prosthesis has complex effects on heart rate and on its variability in humans. Epilepsia 2001; 42:1007–16.

11. Malow BA, Edwards J, Marzec M et al. Effects of vagus nerve stimulation on respiration during sleep: a pilot study. Neurology 2000; 55:1450–4.

12. Asconape JJ, Moore DD, Zipes DP et al. Bradycardia and asystole with the use of vagus nerve stimulation for the treatment of epilepsy: a rare complication of intraoperative device testing. Epilepsia 1999; 40:1452–4.

13. The Vagus Nerve Stimulation Study Group. A randomized controlled trial of chronic vagus nerve stimulation for treatment of medically intractable seizures. Neurology 1995; 45:224–30.

14. Beckstead RM, Norgren R. An autoradiographic examination of the central distribution of the trigeminal, facial, glossopharyngeal, and vagus nerve in the monkey. J Comp Neurol 1979; 184:455–72.

15. Kalia M, Sullivan JM. Brainstem projections of sensory and motor components of the vagus nerve in the rat. J Comp Neurol 1982; 211:248–65.

16. Rhoton AL Jr, O'Leary JL, Ferguson JP. The trigeminal, facial, vagal, and glossopharyngeal nerves in the monkey. Arch Neurol 1966; 14:530–40.

17. Baracco IR (ed.). Nucleus of the Solitary Tract. (CRC Press: Boca Raton, FL, 1994.)

18. Benarroch EE. Central Autonomic Network: Functional Organization and Clinical Correlations. (Futura: Armonk, NY, 1997.)

19. Menetrey D, Basbaum AI. Spinal and trigeminal projections to the nucleus of the solitary tract: a possible substrate for

somatovisceral and viscerovisceral reflex activation. J Comp Neurol 1987; 255:439–50.

20. Somana R, Walberg F. Cerebellar afferents from the nucleus of the solitary tract. Neurosci Lett 1979; 11:41–7.

21. Rutecki P. Anatomical, physiological, and theoretical basis for the antiepileptic effect of vagus nerve stimulation. Epilepsia 1990; 31(Suppl 2):S1–S6.

22. Kirchner A, Birklein F, Stefan H, Handwerker HO. Left vagus nerve stimulation suppresses experimentally induced pain. Neurology 2000; 55:1167–71.

23. Saper CB. Diffuse cortical projection systems: anatomical organization and role in cortical function. In: (Plum F, ed.) Handbook of Physiology: The Nervous System. V. (American Physiological Society: Bethesda, 1987) 169–210.

24. Aston-Jones G, Shipley MT, Chouvet G et al. Afferent regulation of locus coeruleus neurons: anatomy, physiology and pharmacology. Prog Brain Res 1991; 88:47–75.

25. Browning RA, Wang C, Faingold CL. Effect of norepinephrine depletion on audiogenic-like seizures elicited by microinfusion of an excitant amino acid into the inferior colliculus of normal rats. Exp Neurol 1991; 112:200–5.

26. Dailey JW, Yan QS, Adams-Curtis LE et al. Neurochemical correlates of antiepileptic drugs in the genetically epilepsy-prone rat (GEPR). Life Sci 1996; 58:259–66.

27. Krahl SE, Senanayake SS, Handforth A. Seizure suppression by systemic epinephrine is mediated by the vagus nerve. Epilepsy Res 2000; 38:171–5.

28. Stanton PK, Mody I, Zigmond D et al.

Noradrenergic modulation of excitability in acute and chronic model epilepsies. Epilepsy Res 1992; 8(Suppl):321–34.

29. Saper CB, Loewy AD. Efferent connections of the parabrachial nucleus in the rat. Brain Res 1980; 197:291–317.

30. Herbert H, Moga MM, Saper CB. Connections of the parabrachial nucleus with the nucleus of the solitary tract and the medullary reticular formation in the rat. J Comp Neurol 1990; 293:540–80.

31. Cox CL, Huguenard JR, Prince DA. Nucleus reticularis neurons mediate diverse inhibitory effects in thalamus. Proc Natl Acad Sci USA 1997; 94:8854–9.

32. Jones EG. The Thalamus. (Plenum Press: New York, 1985.)

33. Steriade M, McCormick DA, Sejnowski TJ. Thalamocortical oscillations in the sleeping and aroused brain. Science 1993; 262:679–85.

34. Malow BA, Edwards J, Marzec M et al. Vagus nerve stimulation reduces daytime sleepiness in epilepsy patients. Neurology 2001; 57:879–84.

35. Zabara J. Peripheral control of hypersynchronous discharge in epilepsy. Electroencephalogr Clin Neurophysiol 1985; 61:162.

36. Bailey P, Bremer F. A sensory cortical representation of the vagus nerve with a note on the effects of low pressure on the cortical electrogram. J Neurophysiol 1938; 1:405–12.

37. Lothman EW, Bertram EH 3rd, Stringer JL. Functional anatomy of hippocampal seizures. Prog Neurobiol 1991; 37:1–82.

38. Steriade M, Contreras D. Relations between cortical and thalamic cellular events during transition from sleep patterns to paroxysmal activity. J Neurosci 1995; 15:623–42.

39. Engel J Jr, Dichter MA, Schwartzkroin PA. Basic mechanisms of human epilepsy. In: (Engel J Jr, Pedley TA, eds) Epilepsy: A Comprehensive Textbook. (Lippincott-Raven: Philadelphia, 1993) 499–512.

40. Naritoku DK, Terry WJ, Helfert RH. Regional induction of fos immunoreactivity in the brain by anticonvulsant stimulation of the vagus nerve. Epilepsy Res 1995; 22:53–62.

41. Chase MH, Nakamura Y, Clemente CD, Sterman MB. Afferent vagal stimulation: neurographic correlates of induced EEG synchronization and desynchronization. Brain Res 1967; 5:236–49.

42. McLachlan RS. Suppression of interictal spikes and seizures by stimulation of the vagus nerve. Epilepsia 1993; 34:918–23.

43. Zanchetti A, Wang SC, Moruzzi G. The effect of vagal afferent stimulation on the EEG pattern of the cat. Electroencephalogr Clin Neurophysiol 1952; 4:357–61.

44. Woodbury DM, Woodbury JW. Effects of vagal stimulation on experimentally induced seizures in rats. Epilepsia 1990; 31(Suppl 2):S7–S19.

45. Handforth A, Krahl SE. Suppression of harmaline-induced tremor in rats by vagus nerve stimulation. Mov Disord 2001; 16:84–8.

46. Clark KB, Smith DC, Hassert DL et al. Posttraining electrical stimulation of vagal afferents with concomitant vagal efferent inactivation enhances memory storage processes in the rat. Neurobiol Learn Mem 1998; 70:364–73.

47. Clark KB, Naritoku DK, Smith DC et al. Enhanced recognition memory following vagus nerve stimulation in human subjects. Nat Neurosci 1999; 2:94–8.

48. Takaya M, Terry WJ, Naritoku DK. Vagus nerve stimulation induces a sustained anticonvulsant effect. Epilepsia 1996; 37:1111–16.

49. Zabara J. Inhibition of experimental seizures in canines by repetitive vagal stimulation. Epilepsia 1992; 33:1005–12.

50. Lockard JS, Congdon WC, DuCharme LL. Feasibility and safety of vagal stimulation in monkey model. Epilepsia 1990; 31(Suppl 2):S20–S26.

51. Fernández-Guardiola A, Martínez A, Valdés-Cruz A et al. Vagus nerve prolonged stimulation in cats: effects on epileptogenesis (amygdala electrical kindling): behavioral and electrographic changes. Epilepsia 1999; 40:822–9.

52. Krahl SE, Senanayake SS, Handforth A. Destruction of peripheral C-fibers does not alter subsequent vagus nerve stimulation-induced seizure suppression in rats. Epilepsia 2001; 42:586–9.

53. Walker BR, Easton A, Gale K. Regulation of limbic motor seizures by GABA and glutamate transmission in nucleus tractus solitarius. Epilepsia 1999; 40:1051–7.

54. Krahl SE, Clark KB, Smith DC, Browning RA. Locus coeruleus lesions suppress the seizure-attenuating effects of vagus nerve stimulation. Epilepsia 1998; 39:709–14.

55. Hammond EJ, Uthman BM, Reid SA, Wilder BJ. Electrophysiological studies of cervical vagus nerve stimulation in humans: I. EEG effects. Epilepsia 1992; 33:1013–20.

56. Salinsky MC, Burchiel KJ. Vagus nerve stimulation has no effect on awake EEG rhythms in humans. Epilepsia 1993; 34:299–304.

57. Olejniczak PW, Fisch BJ, Carey M et al. The effect of vagus nerve stimulation on epileptiform activity recorded from hippocampal depth electrodes. Epilepsia 2001; 42:423–9.

58. Koo B. EEG changes with vagus nerve stimulation. J Clin Neurophysiol 2001; 18:434–41.

59. Hammond EJ, Uthman BM, Reid SA, Wilder BJ. Electrophysiologic studies of cervical vagus nerve stimulation in humans: II. Evoked potentials. Epilepsia 1992; 33:1021–8.

60. Tougas G, Hudoba P, Fitzpatrick D et al. Cerebral-evoked potential responses following direct vagal and esophageal electrical stimulation in humans. Am J Physiol 1993; 264:G486–G491.

61. Naritoku DK, Morales A, Pencek TL, Winkler D. Chronic vagus nerve stimulation increases the latency of the thalamocortical somatosensory evoked potential. Pacing Clin Electrophysiol 1992; 15:1572–8.

62. Jueptner M, Weiller C. Review: does measurement of regional cerebral blood flow reflect synaptic activity? Implications for PET and fMRI. Neuroimage 1995; 2:148–56.

63. Grafton ST, Mazziotta JC, Woods RP, Phelps ME. Human functional anatomy of visually guided finger movements. Brain 1992; 115:565–87.

64. Burton H, MacLeod AM, Videen TO, Raichle ME. Multiple foci in parietal and frontal cortex activated by rubbing embossed grating patterns across fingerpads: a positron

emission tomographic study in humans. Cereb Cortex 1997; 7:3–17.

65. Fox PT, Burton H, Raichle ME. Mapping human somatosensory cortex with positron emission tomography. J Neurosurg 1987; 67:34–43.

66. Ginsberg MD, Chang JY, Kelley RE et al. Increases in both cerebral glucose utilization and blood flow during execution of a somatosensory task. Ann Neurol 1988; 23:152–60.

67. Henry TR, Buchtel HA, Koeppe RA et al. Absence of normal activation of the left anterior fusiform gyrus during naming in left temporal lobe epilepsy. Neurology 1998; 50:787–90.

68. Rothstein RD, Stecker M, Reivich M et al. Use of positron emission tomography and evoked potentials in the detection of cortical afferents from the gastrointestinal tract. Am J Gastroenterol 1996; 91:2372–6.

69. Henry TR, Bakay RA, Votaw JR et al. Brain blood flow alterations induced by therapeutic vagus nerve stimulation in partial epilepsy: I. Acute effects at high and low levels of stimulation. Epilepsia 1998; 39:983–90.

70. Henry TR, Votaw JR, Pennell PB et al. Acute blood flow changes and efficacy of vagus nerve stimulation in partial epilepsy. Neurology 1999; 52:1166–73.

71. Vonck K, Boon P, Van Laere K et al. Acute single photon emission computed tomographic study of vagus nerve stimulation in refractory epilepsy. Epilepsia 2000; 41:601–9.

72. Bohning DE, Lomarev MP, Denslow S et al. Feasibility of vagus nerve stimulation-synchronized blood oxygenation level-dependent functional MRI. Invest Radiol 2001; 36:470–9.

73. Sucholeiki R, Alsaadi TM, Morris GL 3rd et al. fMRI in patients implanted with a vagal nerve stimulator. Seizure 2002; 11:157–62.

74. Garnett ES, Nahmias C, Scheffel A et al. Regional cerebral blood flow in man manipulated by direct vagal stimulation. Pacing Clin Electrophysiol 1992; 15:1579–80.

75. Henry TR, Votaw JR, Bakay RAE et al. Vagus nerve stimulation-induced cerebral blood flow changes differ in acute and chronic therapy of complex partial seizures. Epilepsia 1998; 39(Suppl 6):92.

76. Ko D, Heck C, Grafton S et al. Vagus nerve stimulation activates central nervous system structures in epileptic patients during PET $H_2{}^{15}O$ blood flow imaging. Neurosurgery 1996; 39:426–31.

77. Newton MR, Berkovic SF, Austin MC et al. Postictal switch in blood flow distribution and temporal lobe seizures. J Neurol Neurosurg Psychiatry 1992; 55:891–4.

78. George R, Salinsky M, Kuzniecky R et al. Vagus nerve stimulation for treatment of partial seizures: 3. Long-term follow-up on first 67 patients exiting a controlled study. First International Vagus Nerve Stimulation Study Group. Epilepsia 1994; 35:637–43.

79. Morris GL 3rd, Mueller WM. Long-term treatment with vagus nerve stimulation in patients with refractory epilepsy. The Vagus Nerve Stimulation Study Group E01–E05. Neurology 1999; 53:1731–5.

80. Hammond EJ, Uthman BM, Wilder BJ et al. Neurochemical effects of vagus nerve stimulation in humans. Brain Res 1992; 583:300–3.

81. Ben-Menachem E, Hamberger A, Hedner T et al. Effects of vagus nerve stimulation on amino acids and other metabolites in the CSF of patients with partial seizures. Epilepsy Res 1995; 20:221–7.

82. White HS. Comparative anticonvulsant and mechanistic profile of the established and newer antiepileptic drugs. Epilepsia 1999; 40(Suppl 5):S2–S10.

Surgical technique in vagus nerve stimulation

Andras A Kemeny

2

Introduction

This chapter aims to help surgeons who are starting to use the technique of vagus nerve stimulation. It should be emphasized that it is not a difficult operation – as can be seen in the video on the supplementary CD-ROM. A good appreciation of the anatomy is essential but most neurosurgeons will be familiar with this from operations on the anterior cervical spine. The first few implantations may take up to 2 hours but after a few cases the operating time should be around 1 hour. Indeed it is important to reduce the operating time in order to keep the risk of infection low.

The operation has been described in various articles.[1–5] Each surgeon has adopted a slightly different technique and the procedure presented here is only one of the possible versions. The operation is usually performed under general anesthesia, which avoids the possibility of an intraoperative seizure compromising the sterile field or causing damage to the vessels, or indeed to the vagus nerve. Occasional cases may be performed as a day-case procedure but an overnight observation is good practice, even though complications are very rare.

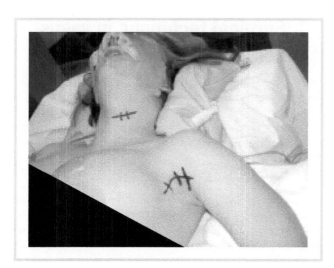

Figure 2.1
Positioning of the patient for the procedure. The recommended site of the incisions is marked.

The considerations of implanting a vagus nerve stimulator are similar to those of inserting shunts or other foreign bodies: the procedure should be done at the beginning of the operating list, with only essential personnel present, and movement around the operating room should be discouraged to minimize the risk of infection. Antibiotic cover is recommended. The layout of the operating room is such that the surgeon stands at the left shoulder of the patient with the scrub nurse to the right and the anesthetic equipment at the foot of the patient. The operating microscope is at the head of the patient. There is usually no need for a surgical assistant to be scrubbed, although an assistant to program the computer and test the device is necessary.

Before the operation starts, the surgeon must establish that the pulse generator is in working order from a communications perspective. The physician information booklet supplied with the device describes how this is done. In brief, after booting-up the programming computer, the generator is placed on the programming wand. The device is then interrogated, the date of insertion and patient code are programmed, and finally a standard test of the device performed. At this stage the generator is still switched to zero output current.

The patient is positioned supine with the neck slightly extended and held by a shoulder roll or suction pillow (Figure 2.1). The neck may be very slightly turned to the right but the straight position may be preferable to avoid the sternocleidomastoid muscle overlying the carotid sheath. The left side of the neck, the left side of the chest to breast level and the left axilla are prepared and toweled up.

The position of the skin incisions for this operation have evolved over the years. The original neck incision was in line with the carotid artery, as practiced for endarterectomy. This was cosmetically unsightly and now almost uniformly a transverse skin crease incision, as practiced for anterior cervical disectomy operations, is utilized. Originally, the incision for the pulse generator was usually placed transversely on the left side of the chest between the clavicle and the nipple. Again for cosmetic reasons, most surgeons now use an incision that is quite lateral, in the anterior axillary fold. Even a technique implanting through a single incision in the neck has been described.[6]

A transverse skin-crease incision is made first on the left side of the neck, at the level of the fifth or sixth cervical vertebra. The dissection is deepened through subcutaneous fat, which is freed from the platysma and retracted with a self-retaining retractor. The platysma is divided vertically, in line with its fibers and with the carotid artery, which should be palpated during dissection.

A second, 'vertical,' self-retaining retractor is positioned at 90° to the first retractor, thus retracting the platysma. This exposes the sternomastoid muscle laterally and the omohyoid muscle caudally, with the trachea

and larynx covered by strap muscles medially. The investing layer of the deep cervical fascia is opened along the anterior border of the sternocleidomastoid muscle, freeing this up. The vertical retractor is then repositioned retracting the sternomastoid. The carotid sheath is then incised in line with the vessels and its edges with the vertical retractor, which is thus placed a little deeper still. It is important to open the sheath in a sufficiently long section in order to allow a suitable length of the nerve to be exposed. This cannot be emphasized enough: difficulties arise in the later stages of the operation almost exclusively only if the exposed nerve is too short.

The upper limit of the exposure will be the common facial vein, which can, if necessary, be ligated. The lower end will be the omohyoid muscle, which can be retracted downwards either with a suture or by repositioning the first, horizontal, self-retaining retractor. Throughout the dissection one encounters branches of the cervical plexus, easily identifiable by their multiple branching. It is usually possible to retract and preserve these.

Within the carotid sheath, the common carotid artery medially and the internal jugular vein laterally are encountered. As described in the anatomy section, the vagus nerve usually lies deep to and in between the common carotid artery and the internal jugular vein. In about 10% of cases, particularly in younger adults or children and in individuals with a thin long neck, the vagus nerve may lie more superficially between and in front of these vessels. One must not easily accept any nerve in this position as the correct one: it may be a finer branch of the cervical plexus following the internal jugular vein. A gentle but thorough search must be carried out in the 'usual' position for the nerve and only when no alternative large nerve is found should one accept an anteriorly placed nerve. If there is a genuine concern about the identity of the nerve, one may consider using one of the intraoperative stimulation techniques described.[7] Usually the artery or the vein, or both, will need some mobilization before the nerve becomes visible. The conventional way to do this is to release the vessels from their areolar tissue and retract them using rubber slings. An alternative method, which the present author favors, is to use the areolar tissue as a 'handle' into which the blades of the self-retaining retractors can be inserted, the vessels are retracted apart without the need for completely dissecting underneath them. This maneuver has been found to be much easier and quicker in the majority of patients by the present author. Naturally, one has to be extremely careful not to injure these vessels and it might be considered safer to use the rubber slings. However, particularly in patients with any sign of atherosclerosis in the carotid artery, too much mobilization of the artery may add further risk.

At this point of the operation the operating microscope is introduced into the field. Once the main trunk of the vagus nerve comes into view, it is gently dissected from the back wall of the carotid sheath. A sufficient amount of connective tissue must be left on the nerve. This allows manipulation of the nerve by holding on to this tissue and will also help to maintain its blood supply: denuding the nerve may lead to ischemic damage or scarring later. However, the nerve has to be freed up from the surrounding tissue over a 3–4 cm length. Most of the time this can be carried out without any hemorrhage. If a small vessel must be divided, it can be cauterized first, using an irrigating bipolar diathermy on low setting. Care must be taken not to divide any small nerve branches following the main trunk of the vagus as these may belong to the cardiac branches. It may facilitate the later maneuvers to place rubber slings or even a thin colored plastic background sheet behind the nerve.[8]

Next the microscope is temporarily removed from the field. The axillary incision is made in the anterior axillary fold, and a pocket is created deep to the subcutaneous fat and superficial to the fascia of the pectoralis muscle, above the breast and below the clavicle. It is usual to dissect about 10 cm medially, approximately accommodating three fingers. This allows the generator to be inserted comfortably in the hollow below the clavicle and sufficiently far from the incision to avoid stretching of the scar or slipping uncomfortably into the axilla. In order to avoid inadvertently injuring vessels in the medial end of this pocket within the subcutaneous fat, one has to see them during dissection. To facilitate this, one of the operating lights can be positioned directly above the chest at this point, 'transilluminating' the skin and fat rather than only trying to shed light into the depth of the wound through the incision. If these vessels are seen, they can be safely cauterized with bipolar diathermy before dividing them.

The tunneling tool is used to create a subcutaneous tract between the two incisions. In the original instructional video supplied by Cyberonics, Inc., it is suggested that it is safer to insert the tunneling device from the cervical towards the axillary incision in order to avoid damage to the vessels in the neck. This may appear so, but the chin of the patient is usually in the way and this may force the tunneling device to enter under the clavicle, thus doing damage at that point. The present author has always inserted the tunneling device from the pectoral end towards the neck, carefully slowing down the forward pushing action when the neck wound is entered. Usually the tip of the device comes through just under the platysma, which is the ideal layer for the electrode. Making a small cut over the tip with a small blade may help the final push. The conical metal tip is grabbed with a pair of artery forceps and the handle rotated to separate it from the tip. After removing the metal rod of the tunneling device, the transparent plastic tube is left behind. The connector pins of the electrode lead are inserted one after another into the tube so that they sit firmly, and then the tube is removed downwards towards the chest incision. This leaves the electrodes under the skin with the ends in the axillary and neck wounds.

The microscope is reintroduced into the field. At this point the surgeon needs one pair of non-toothed forceps in each hand to manipulate the nerve and the electrodes. It may also help to isolate a section of the nerve using two fine silastic or rubber retracting slings, similar to those described for retracting the large vessels. However, it is extremely important not to pull on the nerve by the loops. The helical electrodes are laid down parallel with the nerve, on its medial side and preferably lying just deeper than the nerve. The proximal loop on the lead does not contain the metal strip and it is used only as an anchor, in order to stabilize the electrode and to prevent excessive force from being transmitted to the electrodes during neck movements. Gently lifting up the nerve with one hand, one of the suture ends of this loop is grabbed and pulled under the nerve. Letting go of the nerve, the other end of the suture tail is grasped and the two ends pulled apart, stretching out the coil. Allowing the coil to return to its normal shape over the nerve easily wraps it around the nerve trunk. The residual curl of the coil is gently passed around the nerve whilst holding the thread and the connective tissue of the nerve. This maneuver may sound complicated but it will be very easy to follow if one observes the short video on the CD-ROM supplied with this book. Once this loop is fully in place, it can be gently pushed along the nerve downwards with open forceps, allowing the other two loops to come into view lying medial to and just deep to the nerve. The same maneuver is used to place the other two electrode loops onto the nerve. It is at this stage that the importance of an adequate length of exposure is appreciated: it may be quite difficult to place the third loop on the nerve if this has not been done. Once the electrode is placed on the nerve (Figure 2.2), it will have to be fixed in such a way that allows free movements of the head and neck without tugging on the wire. As was described above, the terminal few centimeters of the lead is finer than the main bulk of the lead, which has thicker insulation. This fine part is now laid as a relief loop next to the nerve and the thicker part held with the forceps in the left hand whilst the vertical retractor is removed from the wound. This allows the large vessels to return to their original position, covering the nerve and the electrodes. A further 3–4 cm of the lead is pulled back up into the cervical wound and this second relief loop is laid either under the platysma or between the

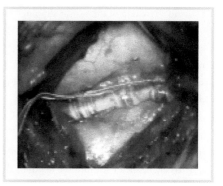

Figure 2.2
The position of the electrode loops on the vagus nerve. The caudal loop is the anchor, containing no metal contact strip (left). The other two loops contain the bipolar contacts (middle and right). The internal carotid artery is lying medially (towards the top of the picture).

platysma and the skin. It may provide a better cosmetic result to place this loop deep to the platysma, particularly if the subcutaneous fat layer is thin. The lead is then fixed with at least two of the silastic tie-downs supplied. The present author usually rounds off the sharp corners of these tie-downs with a pair of scissors before placing them around the lead in order to minimize the risk of them perforating the skin, particularly in children. The sleeves are fixed with non-absorbable sutures to a convenient point in the connective tissue of the neck. The neck wound is closed in layers in the usual manner, with careful attention to a good cosmetic result.

In the lower wound the connector pins are wiped clean of blood and lubricated using the oil supplied with the device. The pins are then inserted into the sockets on the side of the generator (Figure 2.3). The correct polarity must be observed: the connector pin with the serial number and a white marker goes into the socket marked with a positive sign. The watertight seal can cause some back pressure against the connector pin as it is inserted into the generator. This is important because the pressure may push the connector pins out a little. To allow for release of the back pressure, the torque wrench should be inserted before the lead is inserted. The pin must be pushed back in before the screw is tightened and if necessary this maneuver may be repeated. If the connector pin is not fully inserted, there

will be increased resistance that may lead to an early exhaustion of the battery. The screwdriver has a built-in torque wrench, which prevents overtightening of the screws. It is important to insert the screwdriver very firmly into the head of the screws to avoid damaging them while tightening. (It may be prudent to have an Accessory Pack available in the operating room – these packs contain replacement screws and cost much less than a new generator.)

It is now necessary to check the electrical connections of the whole system, as well as the integrity of the lead. This is performed using the so-called 'lead test' in the computer program. The programming wand is placed into a sterile bag, e.g. one of those used for ultrasound probes, and held over the

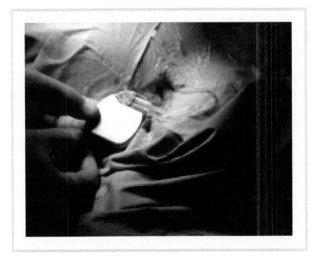

Figure 2.3
The generator (Model 101) is connected to the lead in the axillary wound.

generator. During the lead test the generator delivers 1 mA output current at 20 Hz with a pulse width of 500 microseconds and measures the impedance. No absolute figures are given but the program would return a 'High' impedance message if, for example, there was discontinuity in the lead. This may necessitate replacement of the entire lead with a new one.

Profound bradycardia requiring atropine during this test has been observed (see below),[9–10] although it appears to be extremely rare. If this situation is encountered, one must examine whether the electrodes were erroneously placed around the cardiac branches of the vagus nerve rather than its main trunk. Once the heart rate settles, the procedure can continue.

At this point the present author usually switches on the device (0.25 mA, 5 minutes off, and 30 seconds on) while the patient is still on the operating table. The aim of this early stimulation is to give reassurance to the surgeon, the patient and his/her family that the device is in full working order as soon as the patient recovers from the anesthetic. It also allows a more rapid ramp-up process, as the patient becomes familiar with the sensation of stimulation sooner. Other surgeons inactivate the device by turning the output current to zero. The rationale behind doing so, and keeping a waiting period of 1–2 weeks postoperatively before the stimulator is turned on, is to allow any postoperative edema of the nerve to settle. So far, no ill effects have been observed by the author.

Finally, the generator is inserted into the subcutaneous pocket on the chest wall. It is secured to the fascia of the pectoralis muscle with a non-absorbable suture, using the small suture hole on the side of the generator. Care must be taken to ensure that the excess lead is positioned so that it does not fall between the generator and the axillary skin incision, otherwise it could be damaged when the wound is reopened in the future for generator replacement. Similarly, the lead might be damaged by abrasion if it is placed between the generator and the chest wall. This wound is then closed in multiple layers, again paying attention to achieve good cosmetic results (Figures 2.4–2.6).

Another lead test should be run before breaking the sterile field to confirm the integrity of the system and the correct position of the electrode on the nerve. Finally, the system should be interrogated to ensure that the wand was not removed too early during the lead test as it would leave the output current settings on 1mA.

Pediatric considerations

There are some special surgical considerations when this operation is performed in children.[11,12] The present author tries to avoid the trauma of hospital admission and has performed this operation as a day case in some children who lived locally; they were asked to return the following day to have the wound

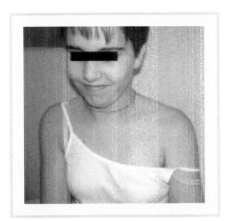

Figure 2.4
The stimulator system is barely visible as a protuberance on the chest wall.

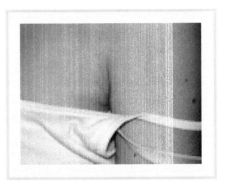

Figure 2.6
Incision in the anterior axillary fold hides the scar.

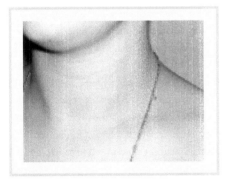

Figure 2.5
The horizontal skin crease incision on the neck offers an excellent cosmetic result.

inspected. The size of the generator, particularly its thickness, may be somewhat of a cosmetic problem in very small children. In these cases even wound closure might be a

problem. One may consider using a tissue expander, as one would for other larger implanted devices, but with all of the present author's cases being over 3 years of age this has not been necessary. The new Model 102 generator is sufficiently thin that it is less of a problem than the old Model 100 or the Model 101. The present author has seen children in whom the generator was placed on the chest wall below, rather than above, the breast; this made the device much less obvious, but when the child grows the lead may become taut, which may necessitate replacing the wire.

The dissection in the neck is easier in children. It is usually easier to find the nerve, and there is much less need to retract the carotid artery and jugular vein. The nerve is thin but its size relative to the vessels is no different to that of an adult, so identification is not a problem. The present author usually uses the same electrodes as in the adult, although different sizes are available. Particular care has to be taken to preserve the platysma and, due to the thin skin, it is usual to try and bury the relief loops under this muscle. The present author had one case, in fact the youngest one, whose skin was penetrated by the sharp corner of the silastic tie-down: since then the corner of the tie-downs have been rounded off to avoid this.

Children can tolerate a much faster ramp-up process, and indeed higher settings, after the operation than adults can. Nevertheless, stimulation is kept at a low level, usually about 1.25–1.5 mA output current.

Complications

Infection

In published trials the highest complication rate was that of infection at either the generator implantation site or the lead implantation site. The overall infection rate was 3% but most were successfully treated with antibiotics and only 1% required removal of the device. In the latest double-blind trial investigating the outcome after vagus nerve stimulator implantation (E05 study), three patients out of 199, i.e. 1.5%, developed infections.[13,14] All required generator removal although in this series one of them was later replaced successfully. In

most of such cases, however, vagus nerve stimulation is usually abandoned in order to minimize the risk of surgical complications during reimplantation. The present author, in a series of 160 patients, has had no overt infection, although the youngest child in the series developed a seroma that required aspiration but yielded no infectious agent.

Vocal cord paresis

Vocal cord dysfunction is a rare complication, which is to some extent surprising, considering the unavoidable manipulation of the vagus nerve and interference with its vascular supply. It may be that the problem arises most in the hands of surgeons inexperienced in the procedure. In an early publication describing 11 patients, two had vocal cord dysfunction.[3] The cause was traced back to the surgical technique: in this case the surgeon tied the suture tails of the electrode together, compressing the nerve and causing edema of it, which was seen during the subsequent urgent removal of the device. Nine months later complete recovery was observed. The remaining patients in that series were then investigated by fluoroscopy and another, asymptomatic, patient with vocal cord dysfunction was found. In unpublished material from Sheffield two out of 160 patients had this complication. In one patient, operated upon very early in the series, there was considerable dysphagia and difficulties drinking liquids. Subsequently, the patient had vocal cord injection with Teflon and showed good initial symptomatic improvement; however, an infective complication to the Teflon injection left the patient with permanent, although moderate, difficulties. The other patient had only a moderate hoarseness of the voice and this was not treated further: the patient continued with vagus nerve stimulation as it resulted in good symptomatic control of their epilepsy. In the E05 study, two subjects (1% of the study) suffered vocal cord paresis.[14]

It is probably possible to reduce the risk of vocal cord dysfunction by careful handling of the vagus nerve. It is self-explanatory that one must not grab the nerve with the forceps whilst dissecting it from the surrounding connective tissue or during the placement of the electrodes. Care must be taken not to extract the nerve too far up from its bed, too sharply or for too long. One must not remove or deplete the vascular supply to the nerve by denuding it from its connective tissue sleeve or through the retraction process. Postoperatively all patients must be observed for any signs of lasting hoarseness or dysphagia, particularly if the patient complains of a cough whilst drinking liquids. The diagnosis can be formally established by video fluoroscopy and swallowing assessment. Most patients require only reassurance if a mild abnormality is reported and in these cases it may well be prudent to wait until the

difficulty is resolved before the stimulator setting is ramped up.

Some patients complain of swallowing difficulties only when the stimulator is turned up to a high output current or turned up too fast. In these cases it is usually sufficient to reduce the setting until the symptom is resolved. Subsequently, as the patients develop a tolerance to the higher output current, the setting can be adjusted again.

Other nerve lesions

Horner's syndrome has also been observed after this procedure.[14] This complication is well-recognized following carotid endarterectomy as a result of damage to the sympathetic plexus within the carotid sheath or damage to the sympathetic fibers in the wall of the internal carotid artery. Minimizing dissection around the vessel is probably beneficial.

Two patients were described, one each in the E03 and E05 studies, who developed temporary lower facial weakness after the operation. It is likely that high surgical incisions were the cause, compromising the lower branches of the facial nerve during dissection.

Bradycardia and asystole

Normally one does not observe any alteration in heart rate either during the operation or during subsequent activation of the vagus nerve stimulator. A very rare, but certainly worrying complication during insertion of the stimulator is an extreme slowing of heart rate and even asystole. Only a handful of cases have been formally reported[9,10] and a few more have been described anecdotally. All these events occurred during the lead test during surgery, which is designed to check the integrity of the stimulator system. During the lead test, without prior low-output stimulation, a 1 mA output current is delivered onto the nerve while the impedance of the wire is measured. Awake patients normally tolerate this output current only several weeks after the operation, so one may consider it a rather sudden strong stimulus. This setting cannot be changed within the software. It is interesting that in some of the cases the surgeons described 'atypical anatomy of the vagus nerve,' including the 'anterior location' of the nerve within the carotid sheath, raising the possibility of aberrant cardiac branches in these patients. To date, no harm has come to any of these patients and the slowing of the heart rate resolved spontaneously or with atropine. Considering the number of vagus nerve stimulation operations carried out around the world, the incidence of such intraoperative asystole is no more than 0.1%.

Wound hematoma

Careful hemostasis should prevent blood clots around the stimulator. The theoretical risk areas are the deepest points of the chest wall incision, where a vessel may not be fully secured during dissection, and of course the large vessels or their branches in the neck may be injured, which may manifest as problems later.

Lead breakage

In the early days of neurostimulation, metal fatigue often caused a discontinuity in the leads; improved choice of metals and better manufacturing techniques have reduced the frequency of this complication. Surgical techniques have also concentrated on pertinent details, e.g. the placement of electrode leads without sharp bends, particularly next to sutures or plastic sleeves holding the wire. The same observations were made with vagus nerve stimulators. Since the lead has been modified, breakage has become a rare occurrence. According to the manufacturer, there were six lead breakages out of the first 4900 implants after Food and Drug Administration approval (a lead breakage rate of 0.12%). Analysis of these cases revealed some technical error during surgery, e.g. omitting the use of a strain-relief loop or placing a suture directly onto the wire rather than using the Silastic sleeve provided. The present author had one case of a patient tripping and exposing the neck to a violent jarring but as the device was working quite efficiently to reduce her seizures, she was keen to have it replaced. Subsequently, the lead was removed and a new one inserted. In another case no precipitating factor was recognized (see below).

It seems that the usual presentation of these patients is an abrupt cessation of stimulation. Whereas it is noticed fairly quickly due to lack of hoarse voice on stimulation, deterioration of seizure control is observed usually over the course of 2–3 months. Regular testing of the device using the magnet supplied allows this complication to be detected at an early stage. This is important, as after several months without stimulation, when the device is turned on again, it may take even longer to return to the previously achieved seizure control.

Replacement techniques

Replacement of the generator

The battery life of the Model 100 was estimated to be between 3 and 5 years, although in the present author's clinical experience it has usually been closer to 3 years. The Model 101 is projected to last for 8–12 years, depending on the settings required for clinical efficacy. As most patients who have a working pulse generator experience some sensation in the throat, or at least their voice

becomes hoarse, when the stimulator is activated, they or their carers usually notice when these effects are no longer present. More importantly, seizure control usually starts to deteriorate.

When the battery is depleted, it requires replacement. This can be carried out very easily. The present author favors this operation being performed under a short general anesthetic because the patient may have a seizure during the procedure. However, as it takes a short time, approximately 10–15 minutes, some may choose to use local anesthetic.

With the patient supine, the old scar on the chest wall is opened. Using sharp dissection down on to the generator the device can be very easily found. The hard casing allows an easy approach, particularly if care was taken during the primary operation not to allow the excess wire to fall between the skin incision and the generator. There is usually a firm, although not very thick, capsule of scar tissue around the generator and this is divided with scissors to allow externalization of the generator. One must be careful not to cut the lead while replacing the generator. It is helpful during this maneuver to palpate the wound in order to make sure that the lead does not get divided. Once the device is lifted out of the wound the generator is disconnected using the hexagonal-tipped screwdriver. The new generator is connected in the manner described previously. It is helpful and informative to test the impedance of the wire, as it gives information about the level of scarring at the top end around the nerve as well as proving the integrity of the lead before the procedure is completed. The generator is now inserted into the pre-existing pocket and the wound closed in layers in the manner described above. It is the present author's practice to carry out a ramp-up procedure during the postoperative period, similar to that after the primary operation, because patients may have tolerance to only a much lower setting than before a break from regular stimulation.

Lead removal and reimplantation

Espinosa et al[15] reported 10 patients who had their electrode removed: these procedures were performed because of lead breakage in some cases and because the device was not effective in others. Espinosa et al[15] found the removal easy even when the lead had been in situ for 7 years. The present author's experience in removing leads in two cases is quite different, the operations being quite laborious. Both cases were undertaken after lead breakage in patients who had had excellent responses to vagus nerve stimulation. Particular care had to be taken to minimize damage to the nerve and to allow reimplantation. It has been suggested that lead breakage could be the result of an earlier design of the lead. However, both of these

cases had contemporary electrodes, so even with these the possibility of lead breakage exists.

Removal or replacement of a lead is done under general anesthesia and the procedure is aided by the use of an operating microscope. Before the operation starts, one has to consult the original operation notes as to whether the relief loop of the wire was entirely buried under the platysma or placed more superficially between the platysma and the subcutaneous fat. Having opened the old incision, one of the silastic tie-downs is usually palpable, even through the platysma. This allows identification of the lead and to follow it toward the carotid artery. Within the deep fibrotic tissue it may not be very easy to palpate the artery and repeated attempts should be made to identify it for safe dissection. The nerve is usually identified only by following the electrode. It is gently dissected out of its fibrotic sheath, ensuring exposure of a sufficient length of the nerve, as in the primary operation. A thin layer of scar tissue still surrounds the nerve and the electrode loops, and the whole complex can be mobilized using vessel loops. At this point, high magnification and the use of microsurgical techniques are essential. Some of the spirals of the helical electrode may fall away easily from the nerve as soon as the fibrotic sheath around them is gently divided using a sharp blade or tenotomy scissors. It has been tried to remove the lead intact in order to allow analysis of the point of breakage but it was found difficult to maintain its integrity, particularly here. Indeed, it is easier to cut the helical electrode and remove it in pieces. The chest incision is then reopened and the generator externalized. After disconnection of the lead from the generator, using the hexagonal screwdriver, the lead can be pulled out very easily. Some sharp dissection may be required to free the wire from the scar tissue between the pectoralis fascia and the subcutaneous fat.

There is usually a series of thicker scar tissue cuffs around the nerve over the sections between the electrode loops, giving it a beaded appearance. It is probably best to replace the new electrode coils into the same sections of the nerve where the old loops were, because removal of more scar than absolutely necessary may lead to damage of the nerve. Naturally, if the dissection is easy, one may try to remove the scar tissue in order to minimize the impedance between the contact points of the electrodes and the nerve. It has been suggested that further dissection towards the cranial base is helpful and this may be borne in mind if one runs into difficulty at the previous operation site.

Summary

Since the original description of implanting vagus nerve stimulators by Reid,[4] more than 17,000 operations have been carried out

throughout the world.[16] The technique has evolved in some ways, particularly with the use of more cosmetic incisions. Technical advances, e.g. more compact and longer lasting new generators and more durable electrodes, have been helpful in making these devices more practical. Careful surgical technique, and familiarity with the anatomy and the device itself ensures low rates of complications. Replacement of the generator after battery exhaustion is a very easy procedure, although it will be less frequently needed with the improved lifespan of the device (up to 12 years). Replacement of a broken wire is possible, although the removal of the electrode from around the nerve can be difficult, raising the option of leaving the lead in place even when the generator is removed due to lack of efficacy. In cases of lead failure where the stimulator has been efficacious this is not an option, and successful reimplantation has been performed.

References

1. Amar AP, Heck CN, Levy ML et al. An institutional experience with cervical vagus nerve trunk stimulation for medically refractory epilepsy: rationale, technique, and outcome. Neurosurgery 1998; 43:1265–80.

2. Bruce DA. Implantation of a vagus nerve stimulator for refractory partial seizures: surgical outcomes of 454 study patients. Epilepsia 1998; 39:92–3.

3. Landy HJ, Ramsay ER, Slater J et al. Vagus nerve stimulation for complex partial seizures:

surgical technique, safety and efficacy. J
Neurosurgery 1993; 78:26–31.

4. Reid SA. Surgical technique for implantation
of the neurocybernetic prosthesis. Epilepsia
1990; 31:S38–S39.

5. Uthman BM, Wilder BJ, Penry JK et al.
Treatment of epilepsy by stimulation of the
vagus nerve. Neurology 1993; 43:1338–45.

6. Patil A, Chand A, Andrews R. Single incision
for implanting a vagal nerve stimulator system
(VNSS): technical note. Surg Neurol 2001;
55:103–5.

7. Vaughn BV, Bernard E, Lannon S et al.
Intraoperative methods for confirmation of
correct placement of the vagus nerve
stimulator. Epileptic Dis 2001; 3:75–8.

8. DeGiorgio CM, Amar A, Apuzzo
MLJ. Surgical anatomy, implantation
technique, and operative complications. In:
(Schachter SC, Schmidt D, eds) Vagus Nerve
Stimulation. (Martin Dunitz Ltd: London,
2000.)

9. Asconape JJ, Moore DD, Zipes DP et al.
Bradycardia and asystole with the use of vagus
nerve stimulation for the treatment of
epilepsy: a rare complication of intraoperative
device testing. Epilepsia 1999; 40:1452–4.

10. Tatum WO 4th, Moore DB, Stecker MM et
al. Ventricular asystole during vagus nerve

stimulation for epilepsy in humans.
Neurology 1999; 52:1267–9.

11. Helmers SL, Wheless JW, Frost M et al.
Vagus nerve stimulation therapy in pediatric
patients with refractory epilepsy: restrospective
study. J Child Neurol 2001; 16:843–8.

12. Valencia I, Holder DL, Helmers SL et al.
Vagus nerve stimulation in pediatric epilepsy:
a review. Pediatr Neurol 2001; 25:368–76.

13. Morris GL 3rd, Mueller WM. Long-term
treatment with vagus nerve stimulation in
patients with refractory epilepsy. The Vagus
Nerve Stimulation Study Group E01–E05.
Neurology 1999; 53:1731–5 (erratum appears
in Neurology 2000; 54:1712).

14. Kim W, Clancy RR, Liu GT. Horner
syndrome associated with implantation of a
vagus nerve stimulator. Am J Ophthalmol
2001; 131:383–4.

15. Espinosa J, Aiello MT, Naritoku DK.
Revision and removal of stimulating
electrodes following long term therapy with
the vagus nerve stimulator. Surg Neurol 1999;
51:659–64.

16. Handforth A, DeGiorgio CM, Schachter S et
al. Vagus nerve stimulation therapy for partial
onset seizures. A randomized active-control
trial. Neurology 1998; 51:48–55.

Vagus nerve stimulation: efficacy, safety, and tolerability in patients with epilepsy

Steven C Schachter

3

Introduction

Despite the recent availability of numerous new antiepileptic
drugs (AEDs), a significant proportion of patients with
partial-onset seizures either continue to have seizures or
experience unacceptable side effects from pharmacotherapy.[1,2]
In either instance, these patients are unable to function at a
level consistent with their capabilities and therefore have an
unsatisfactory quality of life.

While several non-pharmacological treatments have been
used for the treatment of refractory seizures, including
epilepsy surgery,[3] cerebellar stimulation,[4] thalamic
stimulation,[5] and the ketogenic diet, only epilepsy surgery is
widely considered safe and efficacious. However, some
patients are opposed to having intracranial surgery and others
are not candidates based on the localization of their seizures.

Vagus nerve stimulation (VNS) is the first non-
pharmacological therapy approved for epilepsy. The VNS
Therapy System™ (Cyberonics Inc.), formerly known as the
Neurocybernetic Prosthesis, was approved on July 16, 1997
by the US Food and Drug Administration (FDA) as
adjunctive VNS therapy for adults and adolescents over 12

years of age whose partial-onset seizures are refractory to antiepileptic medications. VNS is also approved in numerous European Union countries for use in reducing the frequency of seizures in patients whose epileptic disorder is dominated by partial seizures, and in Canada for similar patients who do not have adequate seizure control with AED therapy. This chapter reviews the results of adjunctive efficacy studies, and the safety and tolerability profile of VNS in patients with epilepsy.

Efficacy studies in patients

The first patient was treated with VNS in 1988 as part of a pilot, single-blind trial of patients with refractory partial seizures who were not candidates for epilepsy surgery.[6] The first pivotal trial of VNS was the E03 study, a multicenter, double-blind, randomized, parallel, active-control trial of VNS in 114 patients with predominantly partial seizures.[7–10] The second pivotal clinical study was the E05 study, a multicenter, double-blind, randomized, parallel, active-control trial of VNS in 199 patients with complex partial seizures.[11] In 1991, a compassionate-use trial enrolled 124 patients with all types of intractable seizures (the E04 study).[12]

The study designs, as well as the efficacy results, of the E03 and the E05 trials will be discussed in detail. Efficacy for other seizure types and in childhood epilepsies will then be presented.

Add-on, double-blind, active-control, parallel-design trials

Study designs

The E03 and E05 studies were multicenter, blinded, randomized, active-control trials that compared two different VNS stimulation protocols for the treatment of partial-onset seizures: high stimulation (30 Hz, 30 seconds on, 5 minutes off, 500 microseconds pulse width) and low stimulation (1 Hz, 30 seconds on, 90–180 minutes off, 130 microseconds pulse width). When the study was designed, the low-stimulation treatment was felt to be less effective than the high-stimulation treatment.

Study candidates were followed over a 12–16 week prospective baseline period during which seizures were counted and changes in AED dosages were allowed only to maintain appropriate concentrations or in response to drug toxicity (Figure 3.1). Patients who satisfied all inclusion and exclusion criteria were then implanted with the NCP system. Two weeks later, patients were randomized to receive either high or low stimulation (Table 3.1). Over the next 2 weeks, those patients randomized to the high-stimulation group had their generator output current increased as high as could be tolerated, whereas those randomized to the low-stimulation group had the current increased only to the point that stimulation could be perceived. Efficacy was then assessed during

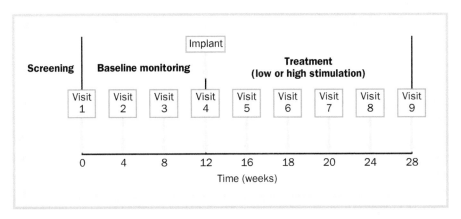

Figure 3.1
Schedule of surgery and visits for E03 and E05 studies.

Table 3.1
Stimulation parameters.

Parameter	High stimulation	Low stimulation
Output current	Up to 3.5 mA	Up to 3.5 mA
Frequency	30 Hz	1 Hz
Pulse width	500 μs	130 μs
On time	30 s	30 s
Off time	5 min	90–180 min

the remaining 12 weeks of the treatment phase. At the conclusion of the study, patients were eligible to enter long-term open studies.

Enrollment information

Patients enrolled in the E03 and E05 studies were at least 12 years of age, had at least six seizures per month, and were taking one to three AEDs. In the E05 study, patients had to have partial seizures with alteration of consciousness to enroll.

In the E03 study, 125 patients were enrolled; 114 completed the prospective baseline and were implanted. The average duration of epilepsy was 23 years for patients in the high-stimulation group ($n = 54$) and 20 years for the low-stimulation group ($n = 60$). Patients in both groups were taking a mean of 2.1 AEDs at study entry.

In the E05 study, 254 patients were entered, including 55 who were discontinued from baseline for failing protocol eligibility: 199 patients were implanted, one patient was not randomized due to device infection, and two randomized patients (one in each treatment group) were excluded from the analysis for administrative reasons. The baseline characteristics for patients in the high-stimulation group ($n = 95$) and those in the low-stimulation ($n = 103$) were similar (Table 3.2), and consistent with the E03 study.

Results

In both studies, the primary efficacy analysis was percentage change in total seizure frequency during treatment relative to baseline, comparing the high- and low-stimulation groups. In the E03 study, the high-stimulation group had a mean reduction in seizure frequency of 24.5%, versus 6.1% for the low-stimulation group ($P = 0.01$). In the E05 study, the mean percentage decreases

in seizure frequency during treatment compared to baseline were 28 and 15% for the high- and low-stimulation groups, respectively. The between-group comparison was statistically significant in favor of high stimulation ($P = 0.039$).

Secondary efficacy measures in both studies showed statistically significant effects in favor of high stimulation. In the E03 study, 31% of patients in the high-stimulation group had at least 50% reduction in seizures compared to 13% of patients in the low-stimulation group ($P = 0.02$). In the E05 study, 11% of patients in the high-stimulation group had a reduction in seizure frequency that was >75%, versus 2% of patients in the low-stimulation group ($P = 0.01$). In addition, both the high- and low-stimulation groups showed a statistically and clinically significant difference in within-group mean percentage change in seizure frequency during treatment compared to baseline ($P < 0.0001$).

Long-term efficacy

There are suggestions that efficacy further improved after the initial 3 month treatment period for patients who completed the E03 and E05 studies, but these results should be interpreted cautiously since ongoing therapy with VNS was unblinded and concomitant AEDs could be adjusted.[9,13,14]

DeGiorgio et al[15] prospectively evaluated 12-month seizure frequencies in patients with

Table 3.2
Characteristics of the patients with medically refractory partial-onset seizures, according to treatment group in the E05 study.

Characteristic	Treatment	
	Low stimulation (n = 103)	**High stimulation (n = 95)**
Age (y)		
Mean ± SD	34.2 ± 10.1	32.1 ± 10.8
Range	15–60	13–54
Gender, n (%)		
Male	44 (42.7)	49 (51.6)
Female	59 (57.3)	46 (48.4)
Race, n (%)		
White	86 (83.5)	85 (89.5)
Hispanic	10 (9.7)	7 (7.4)
Other	7 (6.8)	3 (3.1)
Total seizure frequency per day during baseline		
Median	0.51	0.58
Mean ± SD	0.97 ± 1.13	1.59 ± 3.26
Partial-onset seizures with alteration of awareness per day during baseline		
Median	0.49	0.51
Mean ± SD	0.83 ± 0.94	1.21 ± 1.96
Number of antiepileptic drugs (AED) Mean ± SD		
Taken at time of enrollment	2.1 ± 0.7	2.2 ± 0.7
Previously tried and discontinued	5.7 ± 2.5	5.0 ± 2.3
Years of seizure disorder		
Mean ± SD	23.7 ± 10.8	22.1 ± 11.5
Range	2–52	2–48

medically refractory partial-onset seizures who had completed the E05 study. Patients who were initially randomized to low-stimulation settings and then transitioned to high-stimulation settings as high as could be tolerated for long-term treatment were included in the study. The primary efficacy variable was the percentage change in total seizure frequency at 3 and 12 months compared to the 3 month pre-implantation baseline. The median seizure reductions at 3 and 12 months were 34 and 45%, respectively ($P = 0.0001$, 12 versus 3 months). In addition, one in five patients had at least ≥ 75% reduction in seizure frequency at 12 months. Device changes were not the predominant predictor of increased efficacy after 12 months.[16]

A prospective study of 21 patients (mean duration of epilepsy of 17 years, mean 2.8 AEDs) who were treated with VNS for an average of 13 months showed that reductions in numbers or dosages of AED without loss of seizure control, and with improved patient satisfaction, were possible in 15 patients (71%).[17,18] Interestingly, two out of six patients were able to taper off psychotropic drugs.

Efficacy in other seizure types, and in children and the elderly

Adjunctive VNS may have potential for other seizure types and epilepsy syndromes, including symptomatic generalized epilepsies characterized by mixed generalized seizures.[19] Labar et al[12] reported on 24 patients with medication-resistant generalized epilepsy who had participated in a compassionate-use protocol. Median seizure frequency was reduced by 46% after 3 months of stimulation compared to a 1-month baseline. The best responses to VNS occurred in patients with high baseline seizure rates and later ages of seizure onset.

There are fewer publications of the effectiveness of VNS in children than in adults.[20] In one series of 12 children between the ages of 4 and 16, with medically and surgically refractory seizures who were implanted with the VNS, five patients had > 90% reduction in seizure frequency and four patients were able to reduce the number of AEDs used.[21] In another series of 16 children between the ages of 4 and 19, six children experienced at least a 50% reduction in seizure frequency during the tenth to twelfth month of VNS.[22]

Sixteen children with epileptic encephalopathy were treated with VNS, and were prospectively studied for changes in seizure frequency, electroencephalogram (EEG) tracings, adaptive behavior, quality of life and language performance.[23] One device was explanted due to infection. Of the remaining 15 children, four had at least 50% seizure reduction at 1 year following implant; conversely, two had at least a 50% increase in seizure frequency. Perceived treatment side effects and general behavior were improved, and in six children there was a significant improvement in verbal performance that did not correlate with changes in seizure frequency. Other anecdotal reports in patients with Lennox–Gastaut syndrome (LGS) are encouraging.[24–26]

VNS was studied in 60 children between the ages of 3 and 18 (16 were younger than 12 years of age) with pharmacoresistant epilepsy:

27% of these children had generalized tonic clonic seizures.[27] After 6 months of VNS treatment, the median reduction in seizure frequency was 31% in 55 patients. The corresponding figures at 12 and 18 months were 34% in 51 patients and 42% in 46 patients, respectively. None of the adverse events required discontinuation of stimulation.

Hosain et al[28] studied 13 patients with LGS (age range of 4–44, mean 17 years of age) and found a median seizure rate reduction of 52% during the first 6 months of treatment (range 0–93%; $P = 0.04$). After 6 months of treatment, three patients had > 90% reduction in seizures, two had > 75% reduction and one had > 50% reduction. No patient had a worsening of seizure frequency. Patwardhan et al[29] reported reductions in atonic (80%), absence (65%), complex partial (48%) and generalized tonic–clonic (45%) seizures in an uncontrolled study of 38 children with a median follow-up period of 12 months (range 10–18 months). Other small open studies have suggested efficacy in developmentally disabled or mentally retarded patients with epilepsy.[30]

Sirven et al[31] evaluated the efficacy, safety and tolerability of VNS for refractory epilepsy in 45 adults aged 50 or older.[31] After 3 months of treatment, 12 patients had a > 50% decrease in seizure frequency; at 1 year, 21 of 31 patients had > 50% reduction. Side effects were mild and transient, and quality-of-life

(QOL) scores improved significantly during the first year of treatment.

Efficacy in co-morbid conditions

Clark et al[32] demonstrated that memory storage in rats was enhanced by post-training stimulation of the vagus nerve. Based on these findings, word recognition memory was studied in patients with epilepsy participating in VNS trials.[33] The patients were asked to read paragraphs that contained highlighted words, and then received either VNS or sham stimulation; retention of verbal learning (word recognition) was significantly enhanced by VNS but not sham stimulation. To the authors, the results confirmed the hypothesis that vagus nerve activation modulates memory formation in a similar manner to arousal. The potential clinical application of this work to patients with epilepsy and memory dysfunction is unclear. In another study, 4.5 minutes high-intensity VNS (> 1 mA) on material-specific memory and decision times was evaluated in 11 patients with pharmacoresistant epilepsy.[34] The results indicated reversible deterioration of figural but not verbal memory, and a trend of accelerated decision times during VNS.

Improvements in mood in patients with epilepsy treated with VNS for up to 6 months have been documented in two studies.[35,36] Though different mood scales were used, both studies included adults with long-standing, poorly controlled partial-onset seizures, and in each study AEDs remained constant. In both studies, there was no significant association between seizure reduction and mood improvement, and in one study there was no correlation between 'dose' of the VNS treatment and mood improvement ('dose' was calculated by multiplying the percentage of 'on' time by stimulus intensity).[36]

Hoppe et al[37] used self-report questionnaires, and evaluated changes in mood- and health-related QOL scores following 6 months of VNS treatment in 28 patients whose AED regimen was stable and who had low baseline depression scores. Improvements in tenseness, negative arousal and dysphoria – but not of depression – were observed.

In an open 6-month study of 16 children with LGS ($n = 12$), Doose syndrome ($n = 3$) and myoclonic absence epilepsy ($n = 1$), Aldenkamp et al[38] observed increased independent behavior, mood improvements, and fewer symptoms of pervasive development disorders. These behavioral effects were independent of changes in seizure frequency.

In four out of six patients with hypothalamic hamartomas, Murphy et al[39] reported 'striking' behavioral improvements, including one patient whose episodic rages could be terminated by magnet activation of the generator.

Dodrill and Morris[40] evaluated cognition with the Wonderlic Personnel Test, Digit

Cancellation, Stroop Test and Symbol Digit Modalities Test in 160 patients enrolled in the E05 study. Overall, there were no statistically significant differences in the baseline-to-treatment period between the high- and low-stimulation treatment groups. Similarly, Hoppe et al[41] studied cognition in 36 adult patients before and at least 6 months after implantation using tests of attention, motor functioning, short-term memory, learning and memory, and executive functions. No evidence of cognitive worsening was found.

Malow et al[42] treated 15 patients with VNS who then underwent polysomnography and multiple sleep latency tests. Reduced daytime sleepiness and enhanced rapid eye movement (REM) sleep were noted, even in subjects without reductions in seizure frequency.

Safety and tolerability
Mechanical and electrical safety

Though high-frequency stimulation may be associated with tissue damage,[43] there is no evidence that the vagal stimulation protocols in present clinical use cause damage to the vagus nerve.[44,45] The VNS Therapy system has several built-in safety and tolerability features. In addition, patients may turn off stimulation at any time by keeping the supplied magnet over the generator. This may become necessary if stimulation becomes uncomfortable, or if the patient anticipates a prolonged period of speaking and does not wish to experience hoarseness or voice change from stimulation.

Environmental considerations

The antenna within the generator is controlled by radiofrequency signals transmitted by the programming wand. Nonetheless, neither the generator nor the electrode leads are affected by microwave transmission, cellular phones or airport security systems. Some restrictions do apply to magnetic resonance imaging (MRI) testing, however. Because the heat induced in the electrode leads by a body MRI could theoretically cause local tissue injury, body MRI scans are contraindicated. Head MRI should only be done with transmit and receive head coils; therefore, communication between the treating physician and the radiologist before scans are obtained is essential. Further details are available in the June 2002 Physician's Manual on the supplementary CD, supplied by Cyberonics, Inc., which is also accessible online (www.Cyberonic.com).

Safety and tolerability in the E03 and E05 studies

In the E03 study, safety and tolerability were evaluated with interviews, physical and neurological examinations, vital signs, electrocardiogram rhythm strips, Holter monitoring (in a subset of 28 patients), gastric acid monitoring (in 14 patients), and AED concentrations. Similarly, safety and tolerability were evaluated in the E05 study with interviews, physical and neurological examinations, vital signs, Holter monitoring, pulmonary function tests, standard laboratory tests, and urinalysis.

In the E03 study, the adverse events (AEs; side effects) that occurred in at least 5% of patients in the high-stimulation group during treatment were hoarseness (37%), throat pain (11%), coughing (7%), dyspnea (6%), paresthesia (6%), and muscle pain (6%). Hoarseness was the only AE that was reported significantly more often with high stimulation than with low stimulation (Table 3.3).

In the E05 study, none of the serious AEs that occurred during the treatment phase were judged to be probably or definitely due to VNS. Implantation-related AEs all resolved and included left vocal cord paralysis (two patients), lower facial muscle paresis (two patients), and pain and fluid accumulation over the generator requiring aspiration (one patient). The perioperative AEs that were reported ≥ 10% of patients included pain (29%), coughing (14%), voice alteration (13%), chest pain (12%), and nausea (10%). Following randomization, the AEs that were reported by patients in the high-stimulation group at some time during treatment that were significantly increased compared to baseline were voice alteration/hoarseness,

Table 3.3
Adverse effects of vagus nerve stimulation occurring in at least 5% of patients in the E03 study.

	High	Low	p value*
Hoarseness/voice change†	37.2%	13.3%	<0.01
Throat pain†	11.1%	11.7%	1.00
Coughing†	7.4%	8.3%	1.00
Dyspnea†	5.6%	1.7%	0.34
Paresthesia†	5.6%	3.3%	0.67
Muscle pain†	5.6%	1.7%	0.34
Headache	1.8%	8.3%	0.21

* Fisher's exact test.
†Adverse effects reported only during the stimulation burst.

cough, throat pain, non-specific pain, dyspnea, paresthesia, dyspepsia, vomiting and infection. The only two AEs that occurred significantly more often in the high-stimulation group than in the low-stimulation group were dyspnea and voice alteration (Table 3.4). AEs in both treatment groups were rated as mild or moderate 99% of the time. There were no cognitive, sedative, visual, affective, or coordination side effects. No significant changes in Holter monitoring or pulmonary function tests were noted. Two E05 patients had VNS discontinued during treatment. One patient in the high-stimulation group had two episodes of Cheyne-Stokes respirations post-ictally; after the device was deactivated, two more episodes were reported and the patient's mother requested that the device be reactivated. One patient in the low-stimulation group had the device deactivated due to a group of symptoms that the patient had experienced pre-implantation as well as subsequent to device deactivation. No deaths occurred during either study.

Laboratory values

As would be predicted from a non-pharmacological therapy, there were no changes in hematology or common chemistry values in either study. Similarly, changes were not seen with AED concentrations.

Other studies of safety and tolerability

Among a cohort of 444 patients who elected to continue receiving VNS after participating in a clinical study, 97% continued for at least

Table 3.4
Treatment-phase adverse events among patients treated with low or high vagus nerve stimulation in the E05 study.

Adverse event	Low stimulation n = 103	High stimulation n = 95
	n (%)	n (%)
Voice alteration	31 (30.1)	63 (66.3)‡
Cough	44 (42.7)‡	43 (45.3)‡
Pharyngitis	26 (25.2)	33 (34.7)
Pain	31 (30.1)	27 (28.4)
Dyspnea	11 (10.7)	24 (25.3)**
Headache	24 (23.3)	23 (24.2)
Dyspepsia	13 (12.6)	17 (17.9)
Vomiting	14 (13.6)	17 (17.9)
Paresthesia	26 (25.2)‡	17 (17.9)‡
Nausea	21 (20.4)	14 (14.7)
Accidental injury	13 (12.6)	12 (12.6)
Fever	19 (18.4)	11 (11.6)
Infection	12 (11.7)	11 (11.6)

Only adverse events that occurred in more than 10% of high-stimulation patients are listed.
** p = 0.007, between-groups comparison, chi-square test.
† p = 0.001, between-groups comparison, chi-square test.
‡ p = < 0.0001, within-group, McNemar's test for matched pairs with dichotomous outcomes.

1 year, and 85 and 72% continued for at least 2 and 3 years, respectively.[46] The most commonly reported side effects at the end of the first year of VNS were voice alteration (29%) and paresthesia (12%), at the end of 2 years, voice alteration (19%) and cough (6%), and at 3 years, dyspnea (3%).

QOL scores were assessed in 136 adults before VNS initiation and 3 months afterwards in an open study.[47] Responders (≥ 50% seizure reduction) experienced statistically significant improvements in energy, memory, social aspects, mental effects and fear of seizures; non-responders improved in downheartedness and overall QOL. The results suggest a positive effect of VNS on QOL beyond changes in seizure frequency, though a placebo effect could not be completely excluded. One other small study found no QOL improvement in patients with reduced seizures.[48]

The mortality rates and standardized mortality ratios of 1819 patients treated for 3176 person-years with VNS were contrasted with other epilepsy cohorts.[49] These rates and ratios were comparable with those of other young adults with refractory seizures who were not treated with VNS. Additionally, the incidences of definite and probable sudden unexpected death in epilepsy (SUDEP) were 4.1 per 1000 person-years, consistent with other non-VNS epilepsy cohorts. Interestingly, the rate of SUDEP was 5.5 per 1000 over the first 2 years of VNS treatment and 1.7 per 1000 thereafter.

During the implantation procedure, transient asystole lasting up to 20 seconds has been reported in nine patients (0.1% of all implantations) in association with the intraoperative lead test.[50–52] The lead test assesses stimulator functioning and system integrity by turning on the generator briefly at 1.0 mA, 500 microseconds and 20 Hz. Four patients were acutely explanted, the others were chronically stimulated without difficulty. There were no sequelae in any of the patients.

Cardiac arrhythmias attributable to VNS in patients undergoing chronic stimulation have not been described, though Frei and Osorio[53] reported changes in heart rate and heart rate variability in a study of five subjects. In another study, high-strength stimulation produced no observable acute cardiorespiratory effects.[54]

Other isolated complications of VNS continue to be reported, including chronic diarrhea,[55] Horner syndrome,[56] posture-dependent stimulation of the phrenic nerve,[57] worsening of pre-existing obstructive sleep apnea,[58] and exacerbation of pre-implantation dysphoric disorders and psychotic episodes with VNS-associated seizure reduction.[59,60]

On August 27, 2001, in a Safety Alert, Cyberonics, Inc., cautioned against the use of short-wave diathermy, microwave diathermy and therapeutic ultrasound diathermy in patients implanted with the NCP system due to the possibility that the generator or lead could cause thermal tissue damage. At the time of the alert, there had been no reports of injuries related to these modalities in patients treated with VNS. Diagnostic ultrasound was not included in the contraindications.

Six patients from VNS clinical studies and two patients who were implanted post-approval became pregnant while receiving VNS.[61] Five of the pregnancies resulted in full-term, healthy infants, including one pair of twins. There was one spontaneous abortion, one unplanned pregnancy was terminated by an elective abortion, and another pregnancy ended with an elective abortion because of abnormal fetal development that was attributed to AED.

The possible relationship of VNS to swallowing difficulties[22] was studied by barium swallow in a series of eight children.[62] Laryngeal penetration of barium was present in three patients without stimulation and was caused by VNS in one other patient. Results from another small series of children treated with chronic VNS suggest that some children with severe mental and motor retardation who are dependent on assisted feeding may be at increased risk for aspiration while being fed during vagus stimulation.[63]

Clinical use of vagus nerve stimulation (VNS) for epilepsy

Over 17,000 patients have been treated with the VNS Therapy system worldwide. Experience has shown that the successful implementation of a VNS program requires a coordinated team approach to facilitate patient education, surgical implantation and follow-up visits for programming changes.[64]

Clinicians must determine the place of VNS in the growing armamentarium for the treatment of seizures. The successful application of VNS presents three practical problems: (1) there is no measurable physiologic response to VNS with which to individually monitor and adjust stimulation; (2) patient- and epilepsy-related variables that can be used prospectively to identify good candidates for VNS are not yet known; (3) the initial cost is high. These limitations and others have prompted a discussion of the appropriate role of VNS in the treatment of epilepsy.[65] Yet despite these limitations, VNS therapy may be considered reasonable and necessary for patients whose partial-onset seizures adversely affect their QOL, and which cannot be controlled after several trials of appropriate AED, alone or in combination, have failed. The use of VNS in patients with generalized epilepsies at this time is based on open, uncontrolled data, and while the results of those investigations are promising, further controlled studies are warranted. Furthermore,

the high initial cost of VNS treatment is more than offset by reductions in direct medical expenses due to epilepsy within the first 2 years after implantation in some patients.[66]

Some clinicians experienced in the use of VNS alter the 'high'-stimulation protocols used in the E03 and E05 studies if satisfactory seizure reduction is not obtained after 3–6 months of therapy. For example, VNS efficacy may be improved in some patients by reducing the stimulation off time from 5 to 1.8 minutes.[67]

Summary

VNS is effective, safe, and well tolerated in patients with long-standing, refractory partial-onset seizures.[68] The most frequently encountered AEs typically occur during stimulation, are usually mild to moderate in severity, and resolve with reduction in current intensity or spontaneously over time. Conspicuously absent with VNS stimulation therapy are the typical central nervous system side effects of AEDs. There are no apparent effects of VNS on vagally mediated visceral function or AED serum concentrations.

Though the precise mechanism of action of VNS remains unknown, the introduction of effective stimulation therapy for epilepsy has ushered in the non-pharmacological era in the treatment of seizures. The currently available evidence shows that VNS is effective, safe and well tolerated in patients with longstanding, refractory partial-onset seizures, and may be beneficial to patients with other forms of epilepsy, including LGS. Complications from the implantation procedure are infrequent and manageable,[69] and further enhancements in surgical techniques and post-operative care are likely to continue.[70–73] There has been no indication of tolerance to therapeutic effect in long-term, open studies. Accumulating evidence of efficacy for other seizure types, and in children and the elderly, is encouraging.

While relatively few patients with medically resistant epilepsy become seizure free with VNS, there are suggestions in open studies that efficacy, tolerability and QOL further improve over time.[15,18] Given the possibility that the onset of efficacy may be delayed, it is prudent to wait at least 1 year, if not longer, before concluding that VNS has had no effect on seizure frequency or severity. Pending further studies, caution may be warranted when recommending VNS for patients with sleep apnea and cardiac conduction disorders.

The appropriate role of VNS in the treatment of epilepsy remains under active discussion.[74–76] Many epileptologists now consider this therapy an option for patients whose partial-onset seizures adversely affect their QOL, despite trials with three or more AEDs that are appropriate for partial seizures and that have been titrated to maximally tolerated doses, and for patients who do not have surgically remediable partial seizures. The use of VNS in patients with generalized epilepsies at the present time is supported only by open, uncontrolled studies, though results are promising.

The application of VNS therapy will be enhanced once a measurable physiologic response to VNS is identified that can be used to 'titrate' stimulation. In this regard, Koo et al[77] had impressive results in 20 patients when they used EEG findings at 6 months post-implantation, including clustering and synchronization of epileptiform activity, to guide further VNS programming.

Further controlled studies should be performed in patients with generalized seizures and epilepsy syndromes in order to determine: (1) how VNS therapy can be individualized to maximize its effectiveness, either with intermittent stimulation or acutely with the magnet; (2) whether VNS complements AEDs or non-AEDs with particular mechanisms of action; (3) how to prospectively identify patients who are most likely to benefit from VNS; and (4) the efficacy and tolerability of adjunctive VNS compared with adjunctive AED therapy, particularly early in the course of epilepsy.

References

1. Lhatoo SD, Wong IC, Polizzi G, Sander JW. Long-term retention rates of lamotrigine, gabapentin, and topiramate in chronic epilepsy. Epilepsia 2000; 41:1592–6.

2. Fisher RS, Vickrey BG, Gibson P et al. The impact of epilepsy from the patient's perspective II. Views about therapy and health care. Epilepsy Res 2000; 41:53–61.

3. Kemeny AA. Surgery for epilepsy. Seizure 2001; 10:461–5.

4. Loddenkemper T, Pan A, Neme S et al. Deep brain stimulation in epilepsy. J Clin Neurophysiol 2001; 18:514–32.

5. Velasco M, Velasco F, Velasco AL. Centromedian–thalamic and hippocampal electrical stimulation for the control of intractable epileptic seizures. J Clin Neurophysiol 2001; 18:495–513.

6. Penry JK, Dean JC. Prevention of intractable partial seizures by intermittent vagal stimulation in humans: preliminary results. Epilepsia 1990; 31(Suppl 2):S40–S43.

7. Ben-Menachem E, Manon-Espaillat R, Ristanovic R et al. Vagus nerve stimulation for treatment of partial seizures: 1. A controlled study of effect on seizures. Epilepsia 1994; 35:616–26.

8. Ramsay RE, Uthman BM, Augustinsson LE et al. Vagus nerve stimulation of treatment of partial seizures: 2. Safety, side effects, and tolerability. Epilepsia 1994; 35:627–36.

9. George R, Salinsky M, Kuzniecky R et al. Vagus nerve stimulation for treatment of partial seizures: 3. Long-term follow-up on first 67 patients exiting a controlled study. Epilepsia 1994; 35:637–43.

10. The Vagus Nerve Stimulation Study Group. A randomized controlled trial of chronic vagus nerve stimulation for treatment of medically intractable seizures. Neurology 1995; 45:224–30.

11. Handforth A, DeGiorgio CM, Schachter SC et al. Vagus nerve stimulation therapy for partial-onset seizures: a randomized active-control trial. Neurology 1998; 51:48–55.

12. Labar D, Murphy J, Tecoma E. Vagus nerve stimulation for medication-resistant generalized epilepsy. E04 VNS Study Group. Neurology 1999; 52:1510–12.

13. Michael JE, Wegener K, Barnes DW. Vagus nerve stimulation for intractable seizures: one year follow-up. J Neurosci Nurs 1993; 25:362–6.

14. Salinsky MC, Uthman BM, Ristanovic RK et al. Vagus nerve stimulation for the treatment of medically intractable seizures. Results of a 1-year open-extension trial. Arch Neurol 1996; 53:1176–80.

15. DeGiorgio CM, Schachter SC, Handforth A et al. Prospective long-term study of vagus nerve stimulation for the treatment of refractory seizures. Epilepsia 2000; 41:1195–200.

16. DeGiorgio CM, Thompson J, Lewis P et al. Vagus nerve stimulation: analysis of device parameters in 154 patients during the long-term XE5 study. Epilepsia 2001; 42:1017–20.

17. Tatum WO. Vagus nerve stimulation and drug reduction: reply. Neurology 2001; 57:938–9.

18. Tatum WO, Johnson KD, Goff S et al. Vagus nerve stimulation and drug reduction. Neurology 2001; 56:561–3.

19. Rafael H, Moromizato P. Vagus nerve stimulation (VNS) may be useful in treating patients with symptomatic generalized epilepsy. Epilepsia 1998; 39:1018.

20. Hornig G, Murphy JV. Vagal nerve stimulation: updated experience in 60 pediatric patients. Epilepsia 1998; 39(Suppl 6):169.

21. Murphy JV, Hornig G, Schallert G. Left vagal

nerve stimulation in children with refractory epilepsy. Preliminary observations. Arch Neurol 1995; 52:886–9.

22. Lundgren J, Amark P, Blennow G et al. Vagus nerve stimulation in 16 children with refractory epilepsy. Epilepsia 1998; 39:809–13.

23. Parker AP, Polkey CE, Binnie CD et al. Vagal nerve stimulation in epileptic encephalopathies. Pediatrics 1999; 103:778–82.

24. Helmers SL, Al-Jayyousi M, Madsen J. Adjunctive treatment in Lennox–Gastaut syndrome using vagal nerve stimulation. Epilepsia 1998; 39(Suppl 6):169.

25. Murphy JV, Hornig G. Chronic intermittent stimulation of the left vagal nerve in nine children with Lennox–Gastaut syndrome. Epilepsia 1998; 39(Suppl 6):169.

26. Frost M, Gates J, Helmers SL et al. Vagus nerve stimulation in children with refractory seizures associated with Lennox–Gastaut syndrome. Epilepsia 2001; 42:1148–52.

27. Murphy JV. Left vagal nerve stimulation in children with medically refractory epilepsy. The Pediatric VNS Study Group. J Pediatr 1999; 134:563–6.

28. Hosain S, Nikalov B, Harden C et al. Vagus nerve stimulation treatment for Lennox–Gastaut syndrome. J Child Neurol 2000; 15:509–12.

29. Patwardhan RV, Stong B, Bebin EM et al. Efficacy of vagal nerve stimulation in children with medically refractory epilepsy. Neurosurgery 2000; 47:1353–8.

30. Andriola MR, Vitale SA. Vagus nerve stimulation in the developmentally disabled. Epilepsy Behav 2001; 2:129–34.

31. Sirven JI, Sperling M, Naritoku D et al.

Vagus nerve stimulation therapy for epilepsy in older adults. Neurology 2000; 54:1179–82.

32. Clark KB, Smith DC, Hassert DL et al. Posttraining electrical stimulation of vagal afferents with concomitant vagal efferent inactivation enhances memory storage processes in the rat. Neurobiol Learn Mem 1998; 70:364–73.

33. Clark KB, Naritoku DK, Smith DC et al. Enhanced recognition memory following vagus nerve stimulation in human subjects. Nat Neurosci 1999; 2:94–8.

34. Helmstaedter C, Hoppe C, Elger CE. Memory alterations during acute high-intensity vagus nerve stimulation. Epilepsy Res 2001; 47:37–42.

35. Elger G, Hoppe C, Falkai P et al. Vagus nerve stimulation is associated with mood improvements in epilepsy patients. Epilepsy Res 2000; 42:203–10.

36. Harden CL, Pulver MC, Ravdin LD et al. A pilot study of mood in epilepsy patients treated with vagus nerve stimulation. Epilepsy Behav 2000; 1:93–9.

37. Hoppe C, Helmstaedter C, Scherrmann J, Elger CE. Self-reported mood changes following 6 months of vagus nerve stimulation in epilepsy patients. Epilepsy Behav 2001; 2:335–42.

38. Aldenkamp AP, Van de Veerdonk SHA, Majoie HJM et al. Effects of 6 months of treatment with vagus nerve stimulation on behavior in children with Lennox–Gastaut syndrome in an open clinical and nonrandomized study. Epilepsy Behav 2001; 2:343–50.

39. Murphy JV, Wheless JW, Schmoll CM. Left vagal nerve stimulation in six patients with hypothalamic hamartomas. Pediatr Neurol 2000; 23:167–8.

40. Dodrill CB, Morris GL. Effects of vagal nerve stimulation on cognition and quality of life in epilepsy. Epilepsy Behav 2001; 2:46–53.

41. Hoppe C, Helmstaedter C, Scherrmann J, Elger CE. No evidence for cognitive side effects after 6 months of vagus nerve stimulation in epilepsy patients. Epilepsy Behav 2001; 2:351–6.

42. Malow BA, Edwards J, Marzec M et al. Vagus nerve stimulation reduces daytime sleepiness in epilepsy patients. Neurology 2001; 57:879–84.

43. Terry RS, Tarver WB, Zabara J. The implantable neurocybernetic prosthesis system. Pacing Clin Electrophysiol 1991; 14:86–93.

44. Agnew WF, McCreery DB. Considerations for safety with chronically implanted nerve electrodes. Epilepsia 1990; 31(Suppl 2):S27–S32.

45. Tarver WB, George RE, Maschino SE et al. Clinical experience with a helical bipolar stimulating lead. Pacing Clin Electrophysiol 1992; 15:1545–56.

46. Morris GL, Mueller WM. Long-term treatment with vagus nerve stimulation in patients with refractory epilepsy. Neurology 1999; 53:1731–5.

47. Cramer JA. Exploration of changes in health-related quality of life after 3 months of vagus nerve stimulation. Epilepsy Behav 2001; 2:460–5.

48. Morrow JI, Bingham E, Craig JJ, Gray WJ. Vagal nerve stimulation in patients with refractory epilepsy. Effect on seizure frequency, severity and quality of life. Seizure 2000; 9:442–5.

49. Annegers JF, Coan SP, Hauser WA, Leestma J. Epilepsy, vagal nerve stimulation by the NCP system, all-cause mortality, and sudden, unexpected, unexplained death. Epilepsia 2000; 41:549–53.

50. Asconape JJ, Moore DD, Zipes DP et al. Bradycardia and asystole with the use of vagus nerve stimulation for the treatment of epilepsy: a rare complication of intraoperative device testing. Epilepsia 1999; 40:1452–4.

51. Tatum WO, Moore DB, Stecker MM et al. Ventricular asystole during vagus nerve stimulation for epilepsy in humans. Neurology 1999; 52:1267–9.

52. Andriola MR, Rosenzweig T, Vlay S. Vagus nerve stimulator (VNS): induction of asystole during implantation with subsequent successful stimulation. Epilepsia 2000; 41(Suppl 7):223.

53. Frei MG, Osorio I. Left vagus nerve stimulation with the Neurocybernetic Prosthesis has complex effects on heart rate and on its variability in humans. Epilepsia 2001; 42:1007–16.

54. Binks AP, Paydarfar D, Schachter SC et al. High strength stimulation of the vagus nerve in awake humans: a lack of cardiorespiratory effects. Respir Physiol 2001; 127:125–33.

55. Sanossian N, Haut S. Chronic diarrhea associated with vagal nerve stimulation. Neurology 2002; 58:330.

56. Kim W, Clancy RR, Liu GT. Horner syndrome associated with implantation of a vagus nerve stimulator. Am J Ophthalmol 2001; 131:383–4.

57. Leijten FSS, Van Rijen PC. Stimulation of the phrenic nerve as a complication of vagus nerve pacing in a patient with epilepsy. Neurology 1998; 51:1224–5.

58. Malow BA, Edwards J, Marzec M et al. Effects of vagus nerve stimulation on

respiration during sleep: a pilot study. Neurology 2000; 55:1450–4.

59. Blumer D, Davies K, Alexander A, Morgan S. Major psychiatric disorders subsequent to treating epilepsy by vagus nerve stimulation. Epilepsy Behav 2001; 2:466–72.

60. Prater JF. Recurrent depression with vagus nerve stimulation. Am J Psychiatry 2001; 158:816–17.

61. Ben-Menachem E, Ristanovic R, Murphy J. Gestational outcomes in patients with epilepsy receiving vagus nerve stimulation. Epilepsia 1998; 39(Suppl 6):180.

62. Schallert G, Foster J, Lindquist N, Murphy JV. Chronic stimulation of the left vagal nerve in children: effect on swallowing. Epilepsia 1998; 39:1113–14.

63. Lundgren J, Ekberg O, Olsson R. Aspiration: a potential complication to vagus nerve stimulation. Epilepsia 1998; 39:998–1000.

64. Doerksen K, Klassen L. Vagus nerve stimulation therapy: nurses role in a collaborative approach to a program. Axone 1998; 20:6–9.

65. McLachlan RS. Vagus nerve stimulation for treatment of seizures? Maybe. Arch Neurol 1998; 55:232–3.

66. Boon P, Vonck K, D'Have M et al. Cost-benefit of vagus nerve stimulation for refractory epilepsy. Acta Neurol Belg 1999; 99:275–80.

67. Naritoku DK, Handforth A, Labar DR, Gilmartin RC. Effects of reducing stimulation intervals on antiepileptic efficacy of vagus nerve stimulation (VNS). Epilepsia 1998; 39(Suppl 6):194.

68. Ben-Menachem E. Vagus nerve stimulation for treatment of seizures? Yes. Arch Neurol 1998; 55:231–2.

69. DeGiorgio CM, Amar A, Apuzzo MLJ. Surgical anatomy, implantation technique, and operative complications. In: (Schachter SC, Schmidt D, eds) Vagus Nerve Stimulation. (Martin Dunitz: London, 2001) 31–50.

70. Patil A-A, Chand A, Andrews R. Single incision for implanting a vagal nerve stimulator system (VNSS): technical note. Surg Neurol 2001; 55:103–5.

71. Vaughn BV, Bernard E, Lannon S et al. Intraoperative methods for confirmation of correct placement of the vagus nerve stimulator. Epileptic Disord 2001; 3:75–8.

72. Ortler M, Luef G, Kofler A et al. Deep wound infection after vagus nerve stimulator implantation: treatment without removal of the device. Epilepsia 2001; 42:133–5.

73. Liporace J, Hucko D, Morrow R et al. Vagal nerve stimulation: adjustments to reduce painful side effects. Neurology 2001; 57:885–6.

74. Chadwick D. Vagal-nerve stimulation for epilepsy. Lancet 2001;357:1726–7.

75. Binnie CD. Vagus nerve stimulation for epilepsy: a review. Seizure 2000; 9:161–9.

76. Schmidt D. Vagus nerve stimulation for the treatment of epilepsy. Epilepsy Behav 2001; 2:S1–S5.

77. Koo BK, Ham SD, Canady A, Sood S. EEG changes with vagus nerve stimulation and clinical application of these changes to determine optimum stimulation parameters. Epilepsia 2000; 41(Suppl 7):226.

Potential mechanisms of action of vagus nerve stimulation for depression

Mark S George, Ziad Nahas, Daryl E Bohning, F Andrew Kozel, Berry Anderson, Jeong-Ho Chae, Xiangbao Li and Qiwen Mu

4

Recent studies in epilepsy patients, as well as those in primarily depressed patients, suggest that vagus nerve stimulation (VNS) has significant and clinically meaningful antidepressant effects, although double-blind data of VNS in primary depression are not yet available. This chapter describes potential mechanisms of action of VNS for depression, which are interpreted in the light of current theories concerning the antidepressant mechanisms of medications and electroconvulsive therapy (ECT). Even at this early stage in the development of VNS as a therapy, neurobiological studies suggest that VNS might work through several putative antidepressant mechanisms, including its role as an anticonvulsant, or its ability to directly modulate limbic structures known to be important in mood regulation. In the near future, a better understanding of how VNS works in the brain will both answer questions about its putative antidepressant mechanisms of action, as well as provide the knowledge about how to deliver VNS in ways that might maximize its antidepressant effects.

Introduction

Vagus nerve stimulation (VNS) has antidepressant effects in

patients with epilepsy, independent of its ability to reduce seizures.[1,2] Moreover, there have been promising, open, acute[3,4] and long-term[5] antidepressant effects found in patients with primary depression who do not have epilepsy, as discussed in Chapter 5. However, there are still no double-blind studies showing acute antidepressant effects in primary depression patients. In this chapter, it is assumed that the VNS antidepressant effects that have been found in epilepsy patients, in both open and double-blind studies, will also emerge in primary depression patients.

What are the potential mechanisms by which VNS relieves symptoms of depression? VNS is relatively unique as a new form of therapy, so research into this question offers the opportunity to improve understanding of the neurobiology of depression as well. This issue of antidepressant mechanisms is, at first glance, a very difficult topic. First, there is incomplete understanding of the pathogenesis of depression in general. The complex chain of events that causes depressive episodes is simply not understood. Second, there is inadequate information about the mechanisms of action of all known antidepressants, despite their use for decades. Thus, VNS is no different from all other antidepressants, i.e. the mechanisms of antidepressant action are not fully understood.

Inadequate understanding of the neurobiology of depression

A full discussion of the brain changes associated with depression is beyond the scope of this chapter (for in-depth discussions see Post and Ballenger[6] and Post[7]). Currently, clinicians diagnose depression using a symptom-based interview and checklist. There is inadequate understanding of disease subtypes or of the pathophysiological changes that cause these symptoms. Many clinicians argue that this symptom-based approach thus lumps many different diseases under the same umbrella term. To emphasize this point, some researchers use the term 'the depressions,' much as 'the epilepsies' refers to a broad group of diseases, all of which have the clinical presentation of a seizure.[8] The clinical depressions are also complex, as they encompass changes in cognition as well as changes in basic brain regulatory systems and stress hormones.[9–14] Moreover, some of the depressions arise following major life stresses, particularly loss or separation from loved ones,[7] while others arise spontaneously, especially later in the disease course.[15,16] Additionally, the depressions involve changes in several neurotransmitters, particularly serotonin,[17] norepinephrine[18] and, to a lesser degree, dopamine,[19] operating in critical brain regions.[20–23] As yet, there is no widely accepted and comprehensive neurobiological pathophysiology of the depressions.

Current theories of the mechanisms of action of major antidepressant treatments

There are different theories of antidepressant mechanisms of action for the current antidepressant treatments. There is no consensus about these mechanisms and they vary widely. Over the past decade, with advances in pharmacology, much attention has focused on serotonin, norepinephrine, and other neurotransmitters. It is now well established that depressive disorders involve changes in these neurotransmitters and the regions they modulate, and that manipulating circulating levels of these neurotransmitters can improve[24] or worsen[25] depression symptoms. However, despite the current popularity of serotonergic theories of depression, it should be remembered that 10 years ago, the nearly universally accepted theory of how pharmacologic agents altered the defects found in depressed patients involved changes in the hypothalamo–pituitary–adrenal (HPA) axis.[12,26,27]

It is important to remember that, in addition to medications, there are other proven somatic antidepressant treatments. The mechanisms of action of these somatic treatments are not well understood either, but their explanations are more varied than those for medications. For example, light therapy for seasonal mood disorders has been shown to be effective in several large, randomized control trials (RCT) comparing light therapy to plausible placebos.[28] Response usually occurs within 2–3 weeks, and the response rate for non-treatment-resistant seasonal affective disorder (SAD) is between 60 and 90%. As is the case for most psychiatric treatments, the basic translational neurobiology behind light therapy for SAD remains elusive, although there are several good mechanistic theories being tested. It is thought that light passes through the lateral geniculate nucleus and then to the suprachiasmatic nucleus, and that this then initiates antidepressant actions.[29,30] In support of the hypothesis that light therapy works by phase-shifting individuals, Terman et al[31] found that the degree of phase advance with morning light was associated with clinical improvement with light therapy in SAD. A different theory about SAD is that the photoperiod in SAD patients is dysregulated. Wehr et al[32] found that SAD patients expand their melatonin duration in the winter, while controls do not. Their results suggest that SAD patients generate a biological signal of change of season that is absent in healthy volunteers. This signal is similar to the signal that mammals use to regulate seasonal changes in their behavior. This finding is consistent with the hypothesis that neural circuits that mediate the effects of seasonal changes in day length on mammalian behavior mediate effects of season and light treatment in

SAD. Sleep deprivation can transiently improve depression, with near-immediate effects. Several imaging studies have shown that this is associated with changes in the activity of the cingulate gyrus.[33–35]

Electroconvulsive therapy (ECT) is the most effective acute antidepressant treatment. As with other treatments, the mechanisms of action of ECT are not known. It is clear that ECT must produce a seizure in order to alleviate depression. However, a seizure alone is not sufficient. The seizure must be induced over the front of the brain, as parietal lobe ECT that produces a generalized seizure has no antidepressant effects.[36] There are several different theories of how ECT works to treat depression. Many have argued that the ECT seizure sets in motion a hormonal cascade, ultimately working through pituitary hormones to regulate mood.[37,38] To date, there has been no consistent hormone or neurotransmitter that fulfills these criteria. Another interesting theory is that ECT invokes natural anticonvulsant changes within the brain, and that these natural anticonvulsant changes result in depression improvement.[39] It is abundantly clear that ECT has an anticonvulsant effect over time. Whether this is related to the antidepressant effect is still a matter of some controversy. With advances in brain imaging, there has been recent attention on the brain regions that ECT affects. Nobler et al[40] initially found, using xenon single photon emission computed tomography (SPECT), that those patients who go on to respond to ECT have a greater reduction in prefrontal blood flow immediately following ECT. There thus appears to be anatomic specificity as to where the ECT stimulus is most needed and is most effective. In more recent work using positron emission tomography (PET), they studied 10 patients immediately before and then 5 days following a course of bilateral ECT.[41] Compared to baseline before treatment, there were widespread areas of decreased metabolism, especially in the frontal and parietal cortex, the anterior cingulate, and the temporal cortex. What is most interesting about these two studies from this group are that those patients who respond best to ECT are those with the greatest decreases in prefrontal cortex blood flow. Thus, ECT seems to be enacting an antidepressant effect with an initial reduction in prefrontal cortex activity. Moreover, even several months following ECT, when patients are doing well and are in remission, their PET scans are focally and globally reduced. ECT, therefore appears to be causing changes in a prefrontal circuit. What is most surprising about these studies is that the effect of ECT is not to restore prefrontal cortex activity to baseline. Rather, paradoxically, ECT seems to be making an abnormal prefrontal cortex even more abnormal, but is still effective in treating depression.

Evidence for and against several potential mechanisms of an antidepressant effect of vagus nerve stimulation (VNS)

The discussion to this point has emphasized that there is a lack of consensus about the underlying pathophysiology of the depressions, and that there are many different mechanisms of action proposed for the currently effective and approved antidepressant treatments. This knowledge now sets the stage for better understanding and interpretation of what is known about VNS. Importantly, any potential VNS antidepressant mechanism of action must account for the known route of entry of VNS into the brain (see Chapter 1 and George et al[42]). Putative VNS antidepressant mechanisms should also be able to explain the relatively slow onset of antidepressant action of VNS, with continued improvement over long time frames such as 1 year. This trend is shown in Figure 4.1. Although there is only a small body of literature comparing VNS to medications over this time frame, it does appear that with VNS there may be relatively small amounts of relapses or tolerance over time. What, then, is happening at a neurobiological level, starting at the vagus nerve and entering the brain, over slow time periods in the depressed patients who respond to VNS?

Neurotransmitters and cerebrospinal fluid (CSF)

Both clinical and animal studies indicate that VNS likely results in changes in serotonin,[43] norepinephrine,[44] gamma-aminobutyric acid (GABA) and glutamate,[45] which are all neurotransmitters implicated in the pathogenesis of major depression. VNS in animals activates the locus coeruleus, the main source of central nervous system (CNS) norepinephrine-containing neuronal cell bodies.[46] In patients with epilepsy, VNS appears to increase 5-hydroxyindoleacetic acid – a metabolite of serotonin.[43] Since many of the currently available therapies are believed to work using the same neurotransmitters (serotonin or norepineprine), VNS might be acting through mechanisms similar to those hypothesized about with antidepressant medications. It was thus surprising that a recent study of CSF changes over time in depression failed to confirm the finding of serotonin metabolite changes in CSF, and instead found significant increases in CSF of homovanillie acid (HVA), a dopamine metabolite.[47] The two studies differed in their study subjects (epilepsy and depression), VNS use parameters and concomitant medications, which might explain the discrepancy. Further studies are needed, but enough data have accumulated to date to conclude that VNS acts on norepinephrine and serotonin systems, and that this may be an important mechanism in explaining VNS antidepressant actions.

With respect to the light therapy and sleep deprivation discussion above, Armitage et al[48] recently found that chronic VNS therapy produced marked changes in sleep electroencephalogram (EEG) data, moving seven depressed women's EEG patterns towards a more normal profile.[48] Thus, VNS may be causing changes in sleep patterns, which may then be acting to improve depression. It is unclear if these findings have any overlap with the literature on sleep deprivation and depression.

Antidepressant effects secondary to anticonvulsant action

A popular theory about ECT is that it invokes natural anticonvulsant cascades that then re-regulate a system and improve depression.[39] Several other anticonvulsant medications,

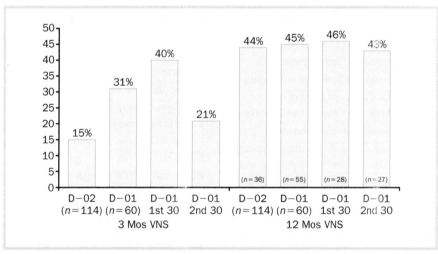

Figure 4.1
Depression long-term response rates in VNS trials. *This bar graph highlights the acute and long-term antidepressant results from the two antidepressant treatment trials. The y-axis represents the percentage of all subjects in the trial who are classified as responders (>50% reduction from baseline in depression symptoms). D–01 was the first open depression treatment trial, which consisted of two cohorts (first 30 subjects, second 30 subjects). D-02 is the recently completed blinded multicenter trial. The D-02 subjects included in this figure are only a portion of the total sample and the follow-up results are derived from a naturalistic, uncontrolled follow-up study. When thinking about vagus nerve stimulation's (VNS) antidepressant mechanism of action, it is important to consider that the antidepressant effects are only modest acutely, but continue to improve up to 1 year or longer. Although there are not a lot of comparable studies with other antidepressants, it appears that VNS effects are different, with long-term improvement and little relapse or tolerance. These clinical data may provide a clue that whatever mechanism or mechanisms VNS is triggering, they must work on a gradual and lengthy time frame.*

including carbamazepine[49] and lamotrigine,[50] also have antidepressant effects, and the anticonvulsant effects of VNS are well established. Thus, it may be that VNS improves depression by manipulating anticonvulsant systems in the brain. Recent work by Dean et al,[51] in epilepsy patients with VNS implanted for 6–12 months, demonstrates the powerful and persistent anticonvulsant effects of VNS. These researchers used transcranial magnetic stimulation (TMS) to study the effects of acute VNS on motor threshold (MT) and the cortical silent period (CSP) following a TMS pulse. These are TMS measures of cortical excitability. Most interestingly, in epilepsy patients who had been receiving TMS for >6 months, there was a significant decrease in motor cortex excitability while VNS was on, compared with 30 minutes following VNS being turned off. However, not all anticonvulsants have antidepressant effects. Further work is needed to understand the mechanisms by which VNS stops seizures, and whether these are the same as or similar to mechanisms working to improve mood in depression.

Changing regional functional anatomy

Structural and functional imaging studies over the past 20 years in emotion regulation[52] and depression[53] have drawn attention to a 'functional neuroanatomy of depression.' One of the current main concepts is that clinical depression arises through an imbalance in prefrontal–limbic circuits (see Figure 4.2). There have been several imaging studies over the past 10 years examining antidepressant treatments and how they cause changes in these circuits. Through the known projections of the vagus nerve, it is clear that VNS could theoretically cause changes in these limbic and orbitofrontal regions. This knowledge was important in justifying the first clinical trials of VNS in depression. Several functional imaging studies with VNS now show that this idea was correct and that VNS, repeatedly and over time, causes changes in these key brain regions.[54]

Studies combining functional brain imaging with VNS offer the promise of elucidating the antidepressant mechanisms of action of VNS. Fast imaging methods like functional magnetic resonance imaging (fMRI) can demonstrate the immediate effects of VNS, while slower imaging methods like SPECT and PET can demonstrate the longer term changes associated with constant VNS over time as a therapy. At the Medical University of South Carolina (MUSC), the present authors have recently succeeded in performing blood oxygen level dependent (BOLD) fMRI studies in depressed patients implanted with VNS as part of an initial pilot study,[3–5] and a more recent, larger double-blind trial. An initial study using the

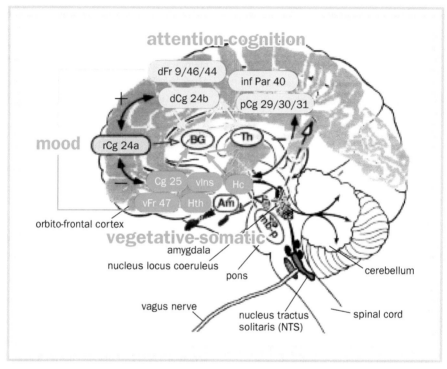

Figure 4.2
Vagus nerve stimulation (VNS) modulates cortical/subcortical systems implicated in mood dysregulation.
This is a midline sagittal drawing of the brain, showing the origin of the VNS signal (bottom), and how that signal then interacts with subcortical and cortical regions involved in mood regulation. VNS sends its initial signals through the NTS, and then to several key subcortical sites, including the locus coeruleus, amygdala, hippocampus, and orbitofrontal cortex. A popular current theory of depression pathogenesis is that depression involves a dysregulated interplay between cortical and subcortical regions. It is clear from the VNS imaging studies to date that VNS sends signals to these important regions. VNS may have antidepressant actions by gradually changing the dynamics of this system over time. (Image courtesy of Dr Ziad Nahas; modified from Mayberg et al[22] and George et al.[42])

interleaved VNS/fMRI technique showed that VNS immediately activates many anterior paralimbic regions, including the orbitofrontal cortex, insula and medial temporal lobe.[55] A follow-up study using the same technique

showed that VNS at 5 Hz had a much smaller brain effect than did VNS at 20 Hz.[56] Most recently, the present authors have serially scanned 17 depressed patients in the DO2 study using the VNS/fMRI interleaved

	Virgin VNS	@ 2 weeks	2w from Virgin	@ 10 weeks	10w from Virgin
Increases	Fronto-temporal* (rt IFG, MFG)	Fronto-temporal** (rt STG, Uncus, Lt MFG, IFG)	Fronto-temporal** (rt STG, MTG, Lt MFG, IFG)	Fronto-temporal* (rt STG, MTG, Uncus, Lt IFG)	– – –
Decreases	Temporal* Lt tempo Rt F precentral gyrus	Limbic* Hippocamp Cbll	Limbic and Posterior** Lt Cbll, Rt Parahippo, Rt O, BA19, SFG	Limbic**** (Lt MFG, BA6, Rt + Lt MFG, Rt cuneus, Parahippo, Lt P	Limbic frontal** Rt MOG, IFG, MFG, P Postcentral gyrus, Ant Cbll

Figure 4.3
Regional brain activity changes in depressed subjects from initiation of vagus nerve stimulation (VNS) over 10 weeks. *This figure highlights the changes observed in an ongoing longitudinal series of VNS functional magnetic resonance imaging (fMRI) scans being conducted at the Medical University of South Carolina in depressed subjects enrolled in the D02 study. In this study, interleaved VNS/fMRI scans were done at the moment of first turning on of the VNS generator (referred to as 'virgin scans'), then again at 2 weeks following device ramp-up, and then again at 10 weeks, following an acute trial. Scans at each time point are then compared with preceding scans to assess what has changed in the brain over a course of VNS. At all time points, acute VNS causes increases in cortical regions, with decreases in limbic regions. The arrows show that the magnitude of these effects changes over time as the brain adapts to the VNS signal. Initially, the cortical increases are subtle, with large limbic decreases. These effects rise and peak at 2 weeks, and then decrease over time. This body of work suggests that VNS is acting over time to modulate and change the dynamics of the system described in Figure 4.2. Virgin VNS: brain activity (BA) compared with (C/W) rest, 1st hr of VNS. At 2 weeks: BA C/W rest after 2 weeks of device on and ramp up of intensity. 2W from Virgin: BA with VNS minus rest at 2 weeks C/W virgin. At 10 weeks: BA with VNS minus rest after an acute course. 10W-virgin: change over time from virgin to following an acute course. IFG, inferior frontal gyrus; MFG, midfrontal gyrus; SFG, superior frontal gyrus; STG, superior temporal gyrus; MTG, mid-temporal gyrus; MOG, mid-orbital gyrus; F, frontal; hippocamp, hippocampus; Cbll, cerebellum; parahippo, parahippocampal gyrus; O, orbitofrontal cortex; BA, brudmann area; P, parietal cortex; rt, right; lt, left.*

technique. Patients were scanned at the first moments when VNS was turned on (labeled 'virgin scans'), and again 2 weeks later after a ramp-up phase where the VNS intensity was increased. Finally, subjects were scanned again with the same technique after 10 weeks of VNS therapy. Figure 4.3 illustrates the immediate effects of VNS, as well as the dynamic effects occurring over time, that emerge from this study. These data are consistent with the notion that repeated daily VNS is causing immediate cortical increases and limbic decreases, and that, over time, these immediate effects are changing as the system changes its dynamic homeostasis.

Further evidence for these VNS effects

have been gathered with PET scans before and after several months of VNS therapy.[57] This study suggests that VNS over 3 months increases resting metabolism (FDG PET) in the orbitofrontal cortex, insula and cingulate gyrus.[57] Thus, functional imaging studies are providing information about the immediate and longer-term changes caused by VNS, and how these are influenced by different VNS use parameters and clinical response.

This prefrontal-limbic neuroanatomical theory of VNS antidepressant mechanisms of action accounts for the known projections and role of the vagus afferents, as well as the very slow and gradual time frame involved in resetting a dynamic system. It should be noted that the antidepressant effects of gamma-knife surgery and other surgical lesion treatments for depression also take up to 6 months to 1 year before reaching peak effect.

Perhaps the most important information for the entire field of VNS as therapy is improved understanding of the different effects of use parameters on VNS brain effects. This information can be partially gathered in animal studies, although it is difficult to implant VNS in small animals, and they then are immobile for most of the day. Figure 4.4 illustrates how interleaving VNS with fMRI can help solve the riddles of how different VNS use parameters differentially affect the brain. This figure is from a just completed study examining whether different pulse widths deliver divergent information to the brain. Future work with this methodology holds promise for rapidly and efficiently refining the > 500,000 different combinations of VNS pulse width, frequency, intensity, train length, and off length.

Stress sensitization

Another important concept in depression pathogenesis is the concept of stress

---

Figure 4.4
Acute vagus nerve stimulation (VNS) effects as a function of use parameters (pulse width). These are BOLD functional magnetic resonance imaging (fMRI) scans from one depressed patient, who was scanned three times on the same day. During each session, all VNS parameters were the same, except the pulse width of the VNS signal, which was changed to 130 milliseconds (left), 250 milliseconds (middle) and 500 milliseconds (right). These are transverse images at three different slices. The orientation is from below, looking up at the brain, with the subject's right on the left side of the figure. Superimposed in color are the brain regions that were significantly (P < 0.05) increased in activity during the VNS signal, compared to the moment just before. Note that the acute effects of VNS in this subject changes as a function of the pulse width, with very little effect at the shortest pulse width, and more with a longer pulse width, sufficient to depolarize axons in the vagus nerve. At the intermediate pulse width, there are acute increases in brain regions known to receive vagus sensory input – the orbitofrontal cortex, the cerebellum, the insula, and the medial and dorsolateral prefrontal cortices. These are also the regions consistently implicated in patients with depression. An important area of research is whether functional imaging such as this might help determine effective antidepressant clinical settings. (From work in progress at the Medical University of South Carolina.)

sensitization. This term applies to the phenomenon where repeated mild stresses, over time, build up to where an animal is sensitized to developing depression. Thus, a single stressful event would not produce depression but repeated daily stresses will.[58-61] Reasoning within this stress sensitization paradigm, one wonders whether VNS might

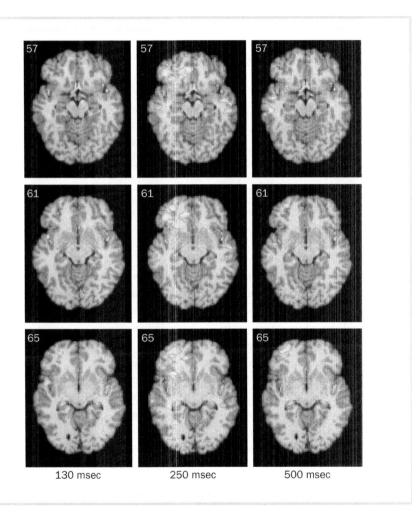

130 msec   250 msec   500 msec

Table 4.1
Vagus nerve stimulation (VNS) antidepressant mechanisms of action.

Mechanistic Antidepressant Theory	VNS?	VNS evidence?
Neurotransmitter Changes	*	CSF 5HIAA changes in epilepsy patients CSF HVA changes in depressed patients
Anticonvulsant	****	VNS is powerful anticonvulsant with chronic and acute changes
Changing Regional Functional Anatomy (Circuits)	****	SPECT changes in depression PET changes in depression Serial fMRI changes in depression
Stress Inoculation	*	Attenuated pain, histamine responses
Hypothalamo-pituitary Axis	*	fMRI studies of hypothalamus activation No studies of cortisol or (DST) in VNS patients

Several leading theories about how antidepressants work are listed on the left. This table then summarizes whether there are studies suggesting VNS might work through these mechanisms. The relative strength of the data is assessed with a 1–4 scale, with modest data (*) or strong supporting data (****). On the right are short descriptions of the relevant studies. DST, dexamethasone suppression test.

be constantly and repeatedly diminishing the abnormal brain reaction to stress inherent in depression. Thus, theoretically, with each new stress that a depressed patient encounters, VNS might be blunting an otherwise amplified pathologic reaction. Then the brain is gradually able to return back to homeostasis without the pathological feedback from repeated stresses. Patients taking serotonin selective reuptake inhibitors (SSRI) commonly report that a stressful life event is no longer as stressful to them as before they were on medications. The present group at MUSC has similarly observed that patients in

VNS depression trials tolerate stressful events much better than before they were receiving VNS. It is thus important to know whether and to what degree VNS might 'stress inoculate' or reduce anxiety, and the pathological overreaction of a depressed individual to a stressful event.

Norepinephrine has long been considered a key neurotransmitter involved in the pathogenesis and regulation of anxiety. VNS, which directly stimulates the locus coeruleus, the primary norepinephrine control site, could theoretically have important effects on anxiety. The historical importance of this pathway that VNS modulates can be seen in the oldest theory about the brain origins of fear, called the James–Lange theory of emotions.[62,63] James [62] and Lange[63] radically argued that all emotion actually resided in the body and it was the brain's interpretation of this signal, through the vagus nerve, that caused someone to be anxious. They argued that, rather than first one becomes anxious, then the heart beats fast and then one gets short of breath, the causal change went the other way. You think you are anxious because your heart beats fast, and then your brain gets a signal (through the vagus) and you experience anxiety. Interestingly, this theory has been hard to disprove and most modern anxiety researchers think that the ultimate answer to the origin of anxiety lies in central-brain-to-peripheral-body feedback loops. However, all agree that the information flowing through the vagus to the brain is likely an important part of anxiety regulation – both afferent and efferent. Moreover, there were strong anti-anxiety effects of VNS seen in a pilot study in depressed subjects;[3] a pilot study is under way of VNS in anxiety disorders. It is thus theoretically possible that the way VNS improves depression is by gradually reducing the downstream effects of stressful life events, thus enabling corrective brain responses over time. This mechanism would account both for the slow onset of antidepressant action, the continued improvement over time and the relatively low

rates of relapse (as stressful events that precipitate relapse are less neurobiologically potent due to VNS regulation).

HPA axis dysregulation

To date, there is no information about whether and to what degree VNS affects serum or urinary cortisol, thyroid function, or other HPA axis measures, such as the DST. Further research is needed.

Summary

In summary, more work is needed to establish whether VNS is an effective antidepressant and, if so, what mechanisms are responsible for causing these changes. From the relatively few studies to date, it appears that VNS could improve depression through several of the current antidepressant mechanism models. There are strong data concerning the anticonvulsant properties of VNS, as well as the changes VNS causes in regional brain activity, both acutely and gradually over time. Because of its unique method of delivery, it may be that VNS produces brain changes through mechanisms not shared by other medications or devices. The next decade should be an exciting one, as these clinical and research studies proceed to understand this most interesting form of brain modulation.

Acknowledgements and disclosure

The authors are supported in part by research grants from NARSAD, the Stanley Foundation, NINDS grant RO1-AG40956, and the Defense Advanced Research Projects Agency (DARPA). The BSL has also received grant support from Cyberonics (VNS) and Neotonus (TMS) for clinical trials. None of the authors have equity or financial conflicts. Drs George and Bohning hold a patent for interleaving TMS with fMRI as a neuroscience tool, and an invention disclosure (with Drs Bohning and Nahas) to use fMRI to determine the optimum treatment settings for VNS. The authors would like to thank Carol Hanback and Minnie Dobbins for administrative help. Dr George would like to acknowledge helpful past discussions with Burke Barrett, formerly of Cyberonics, Inc., and Dr Jake Zabara about VNS research advances.

References

1. Harden CL, Pulver MC, Ravdin LD et al. A pilot study of mood in epilepsy patients treated with vagus nerve stimulation. Epilepsy Behav 2000; 1:93–9.

2. Elger G, Hoppe C, Falkai P et al. Vagus nerve stimulation is associated with mood improvements in epilepsy patients. Epilepsy Res 2000; 42:203–10.

3. Rush AJ, George MS, Sackeim HA et al. Vagus nerve stimulation (VNS) for treatment-resistant depressions: a multicenter study. Biol Psychiatry 2000; 47:276–86.

4. Sackeim HA, Rush AJ, George MS et al. Vagus nerve stimulation (VNS) for treatment-resistant depression: efficacy, side effects and predictors of outcome. Neuropsychopharmacology 2001; 25:713–28.

5. Marangell LB, Rush AJ, George MS et al. Vagus nerve stimulation (VNS) for major depressive episodes: longer-term outcome. Biol Psychiatry 2002; 51:280–7.

6. Post RM, Ballenger JC (eds). Neurobiology of Mood Disorders (Williams & Wilkins: Baltimore, 1984.)

7. Post RM. The transduction of psychosocial stress into the neurobiology of recurrent affective disorder. Am J Psychiatry 1992; 149:999–1010.

8. Georges MS, Post RM, Ketter TA et al. Neural mechanisms of mood disorders. Curr Rev Mood Anxiety Dis 1997; 1:71–83.

9. Holsboer F. Psychiatric implications of altered limbic–hypothalamic–pituitary–adrenocortical activity. Eur Arch Psychiatry Neurol Sci 1989; 238:302–22.

10. Tallal P, McEwen BS. Neuroendocrine effects on brain development and cognition. Psychoneuroendocrinology 1991; 16:67–84.

11. Heim C, Owens MJ, Plotsky PM, Nemeroff CB. Persistent changes in corticotropin-releasing factor systems due to early life stress – relationship to the pathophysiology of major depression and post-traumatic stress disorder. Psychopharmacol Bull 1997; 33:185–92.

12. Rubinow DR, Post RM, Gold PW et al. The relationship between cortisol and clinical phenomenology of affective illness. In: (Post RM, Ballenger JC, eds) Neurobiology of

Mood Disorders. (Williams & Wilkins: Baltimore, 1984) 271–89.

13. Gold PW, Goodwin FK, Chrousos GP. Clinical and biochemical manifestations of depression. Relation to the neurobiology of stress (1). N Engl J Med 1988; 319:348–53.

14. Marangell LB, Ketter TA, George MS et al. Thyroid indices and cerebral metabolism in mood disorders. APA New Res Abs 1994; 187:104 (abstract).

15. Post RM, Ballenger JC. Kindling models for the progressive development of behavioural psychopathology: sensitization to electrical, pharmacological, and psychological stimuli. In: (Van Praag HM, Lader MH, Rafaelsen OJ, Sachar EJ, eds) Handbook of Biological Psychiatry, Part IV. (Marcel-Dekker, Inc.: New York, 1981) 609–51.

16. Post RM, Rubinow DR, Ballenger JC. Conditioning and sensitization in the longitudinal course of affective illness. Br J Psychiatry 1986; 149:191–201.

17. Delgado PL, Miller HL, Salomon RM et al. Tryptophan-depletion challenge in depressed patients treated with desipramine or fluoxetine: implications for the role of serotonin in the mechanisms of antidepressant action. Biol Psychiatry 1999; 46:212–20.

18. Stone EA. Adaptation to stress and brain noradrenergic receptors. Neurosci Biobehav Rev 1983; 7:503–9.

19. Post RM, Rubinow DR, Uhde TW et al. Dopaminergic effects of carbamazepine: relationship to clinical response in affective illness. Arch Gen Psychiatry 1986; 42:392–7.

20. George MS. An introduction to the emerging neuroanatomy of depression. Psychiatric Ann 1994; 24:635–6.

21. Mayberg HS, Brannan SK, Mahurin RK et al.

Cingulate function in depression: a potential predictor of treatment response. NeuroReport 1997; 8:1057–61.

22. Mayberg HS, Liotti M, Brannan SK et al. Reciprocal limbic–cortical function and negative mood: converging PET findings in depression and normal sadness. Am J Psychiatry 1999; 156:675–82.

23. Bremner JD, Innis RB, Salomon RM et al. PET measurement of cerebral metabolic correlates of tryptophan depletion-induced depressive relapse. Arch Gen Psychiatry 1997; 54:364–74.

24. Van Praag HM, Kahn R, Asnis GM et al. Therapeutic indications for serotonin-potentiating compounds: a hypothesis. Biol Psychiatry 1987; 22:205–12.

25. Delgado PL, Charney DS, Price LH et al. Serotonin function and the mechanism of antidepressant action. Reversal of antidepressant-induced remission by rapid depletion of plasma tryptophan. Arch Gen Psychiatry 1990; 47:411–18.

26. Carroll BJ, Feinberg M, Greden JF et al. Diagnosis of endogenous depression. Comparison of clinical, research and neuroendocrine criteria. J Affect Disord 1980; 2:177–94.

27. Arana GW, Baldessarini RJ, Ornsteen M. The dexamethasone suppression test for diagnosis and prognosis in psychiatry. Commentary and review. Arch Gen Psychiatry 1985; 42:1193–204.

28. Terman M, Terman JS, Quitkin FM et al. Light therapy for seasonal affective disorder. A review of efficacy. Neuropsychopharmacol 1989; 2:1–22.

29. Kasper S, Rogers SLB, Yancey A et al. Phototherapy in individuals with and without

subsyndromal seasonal affective disorder. Arch Gen Psychiatry 1989; 46:837–44.

30. Rosenthal NE, Sack DA, Carpenter CJ. Antidepressant effects of light in seasonal affective disorder. Am J Psychiatry 1985; 142:163–70.

31. Terman JS, Terman M, Lo ES, Cooper TB. Circadian time of morning light administration and therapeutic response in winter depression. Arch Gen Psychiatry 2001; 58:69–75.

32. Wehr TA, Duncan WC, Sher L et al. A circadian signal of change of season in patients with seasonal affective disorder. Arch Gen Psychiatry 2001; 58:1108–14.

33. Wu JC, Bunney WE. The biological basis of an antidepressant response to sleep deprivation and relapse: review and hypothesis. Am J Psychiatry 1990; 147:14–21.

34. Wu JC, Gillin JC, Buchsbaum MS et al. Effect of sleep deprivation on brain metabolism of depressed patients. Am J Psychiatry 1992; 149:538–43.

35. Ebert D, Feistel H, Barocka A. Effects of sleep deprivation on the limbic system and the frontal lobes in affective disorders: a study with Tc-99m-HMPAO SPECT. Psychiatry Res 1991; 40:247–51.

36. Sackeim HA, Prudic J, Devanand DP et al. Effects of stimulus intensity and electrode placement on the efficacy and cognitive effects of electroconvulsive therapy. N Engl J Med 1993; 328:839–46.

37. Fink M. How does convulsive therapy work? Neuropsychopharmacology 1990; 3:73–82.

38. Fink M. Theories of the antidepressant efficacy of convulsive therapy (ECT). In: (Post RM, Ballenger JC, eds) Neurobiology of

Mood Disorders. (Williams & Wilkins: Baltimore, 1984) 721–30.

39. Sackeim HA, Decina P, Prohornik S et al. Anticonvulsant and antidepressant properties of electroconvulsive therapy: a proposed mechanism of action. Biol Psychiatry 1983; 18:1301–10.

40. Nobler MS, Sackeim HA, Prohovnik I et al. Regional cerebral blood flow in mood disorders, III. Treatment and clinical response. Arch Gen Psychiatry 1994; 51:884–97.

41. Nobler MS, Oquendo MA, Kegeles LS et al. Decreased regional brain metabolism after ECT. Am J Psychiatry 2001; 158:305–8.

42. George MS, Sackeim HA, Rush AJ et al. Vagus nerve stimulation: a new tool for brain research and therapy. Biol Psychiatry 2000; 47:287–95.

43. Ben-Menachem E, Hamberger A, Hedner T et al. Effects of vagus nerve stimulation on amino acids and other metabolites in the CSF of patients with partial seizures. Epilepsy Res 1995; 20:221–7.

44. Krahl SE, Clark KB, Smith DC, Browning RA. Locus coeruleus lesions suppress the seizure attenuating effects of vagus nerve stimulation. Epilepsia 1998; 39:709–14.

45. Walker BR, Easton A, Gale K. Regulation of limbic motor seizures by GABA and glutamate transmission in nucleus tractus solitarius. Epilepsia 1999; 40:1051–7.

46. Naritoku DK, Terry WJ, Helfert RH. Regional induction of fos immunoreactivity in the brain by anticonvulsant stimulation of the vagus nerve. Epilepsy Res 1995; 22:53–62.

47. Carpenter LL, Moreno F, Kling MA. Effects of vagus nerve stimulation on cerebrospinal

fluid in depressed patients. Biol Psychiatry 2002; 51:152S (abstract 449).

48. Armitage R, Husain M, Hoffman R, Rush AJ. Effects of vagus nerve stimulation on sleep in depressed subjects. Biol Psychiatry 2002; 51:152S (abstract 446).

49. Ballenger JC, Post RM. Carbamazepine in manic-depressive illness: a new treatment. Am J Psychiatry 1980; 137:782–90.

50. Fatemi SH, Rapport DJ, Calabrese JR, Thuras P. Lamotrigine in rapid-cycling bipolar disorder. J Clin Psychiatry 1997; 58:522–7.

51. Dean AC, Wu AT, Burgut FT, Labar DR. Motor cortex excitability in epilepsy patients treated with vagus nerve stimulation. Am Epilepsy Soc Meeting 2002 (abstract).

52. George MS, Ketter TA, Parekh PI et al. Brain activity during transient sadness and happiness in healthy women. Am J Psychol 1995; 152:341–51.

53. Kimbrell TA, Ketter TA, George MS et al. Regional cerebral glucose utilization in patients with a range of severities of unipolar depression. Biol Psychiatry 2002; 51:237–52.

54. Chae JH, Nahas Z, Lomarev M et al. A review of functional neuroimaging studies of vagus nerve stimulation (VNS). J Psychiatr Res 2002 (in press).

55. Bohning DE, Lomarev MP, Denslow S et al. Feasibility of vagus nerve stimulation–synchronized blood oxygenation level-dependent functional MRI. Invest Radiol 2001; 36:470–9.

56. Lomarev M, Denslow S, Nahas Z et al. Vagus nerve stimulation (VNS) synchronized BOLD fMRI suggests that VNS in depressed adults has frequency and/or dose dependent effects at rest and during a simple task. J Psychiatry Res 2002; 36:219–27.

57. Conway CR, Chibnall JT, Li X, George MS. Changes in brain metabolism in response to chronic vagus nerve stimulation in depression. Biol Psychiatry 2002; 51:8S (abstract 544).

58. Molina VA, Volosin M, Cancela L et al. Effect of chronic variable stress on monoamine receptors: influence of imipramine administration. Pharmacol Biochem Behav 1990; 35:335–40.

59. Cole BJ, Cador M, Stinus L et al. Central administration of a CRF antagonist blocks the development of stress-induced behavioral sensitization. Brain Res 1990; 512:343–6.

60. Caggiula AR, Antelman SM, Aul E et al. Prior stress attenuates the analgesic response but sensitizes the corticosterone and cortical dopamine responses to stress 10 days later. Psychopharmacology (Berl) 1989; 99:233–7.

61. Antelman SM, Caggiula AR. Mechanisms of stimulant and stress sensitization: where to look. Clin Neuropharmacol 1990; 13:585–6.

62. James W. What is an emotion? Mind 1884; 9:188–205.

63. Lange C. Ueber Gemuthsbewegungen: Eine Psychophysiologische Studie. (Verlag Von Theodore Thomas: Leipzig, Germany, 1887.)

Vagus nerve stimulation: clinical results in depression

A John Rush

5

Introduction

This chapter briefly reviews the epidemiology, course and risk factors for bipolar and unipolar mood disorders, with particular attention to the risk factors for chronic or recurrent courses of illness. An overview of the acute and longer term treatment issues of unipolar and bipolar disorders is provided. The chapter then summarizes recent research reports of both acute and longer term safety, tolerability and clinical outcomes associated with the use of vagus nerve stimulation (VNS) when added to ongoing medication treatment for outpatients in the treatment of resistant major depressive episodes as part of either non-psychotic major depressive or bipolar disorder.[1-3] The chapter concludes with comments on the potential position of VNS in the treatment plan for depression and the need for additional clinical research.

Overview of depression

Differential diagnosis

The differential diagnosis of clinical depression is shown in Figure 5.1. Mood disorders include both unipolar (e.g. major

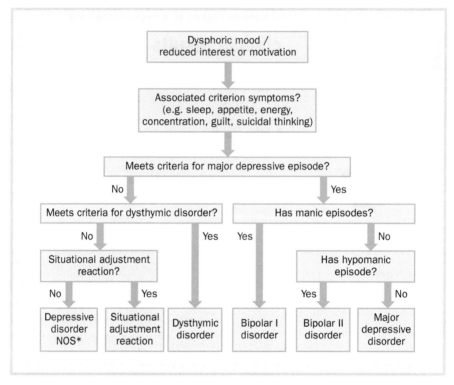

Figure 5.1
Differential diagnosis of depressive disorders not due to substance use or general medical conditions. (Adapted from the Depression Guideline Panel.[14])
*Depression disorder NOS (not otherwise specified) includes premenstrual dysphoric disorders or other so called subthreshold mood disturbances.

depression or dysthymia) and bipolar (e.g. bipolar I or bipolar II) disorders. The latter typically include major depressive episodes (MDE) along with episodes of hypomania or mania. Bipolar I disorder includes MDE and one or more manic episodes. Bipolar II disorder is characterized by MDE accompanied by one or more hypomanic (but not manic) episodes,

though hypomanic episodes may also occur in the course of bipolar I disorder. Major depressive disorder (MDD) refers to the presence of one or more MDEs, without either manic or hypomanic episodes.

Unipolar and bipolar disorders are often severe and disabling with recurrent or chronic courses. They are associated with substantial morbidity and mortality. In such situations, longer term, even lifelong, treatments are recommended.

Dysthymic disorder, another variant of unipolar depression, is characterized as the multiyear presence of significant depressive symptoms and associated disability, during which, for at least the first 2 years, no MDEs are encountered. Over time, dysthymic disorder usually leads to multiple MDEs between which chronic dysthymic symptoms continue. The Diagnostic and Statistical Manual of Mental Disorders, 4th edn (DSM-IV)[4] also recognizes mood disorders due to (i.e. physiologically caused by) general medical conditions (GMCs) (e.g. endocrinopathies, vitamin deficiencies), as well as mood disorders due to substances – either prescribed medications such as steroids or antihypertensives, or illicit substances such as amphetamines, cocaine, or alcohol.

Finally, situational adjustment reactions with depressed mood (e.g. grief reactions) may transiently cause modest disability and a prominently sad mood, along with a few associated depressive symptoms such as appetite or sleep disturbances, impaired concentration, or low energy. The less severe forms of depression may be transient and only modestly disabling (e.g. grief reaction). Even modest levels of depressive symptoms, however, worsen the morbidity and even mortality associated with GMCs such as stroke, diabetes and myocardial infarction.[5–8]

MDD

MDD affects nearly 19 million people in the United States each year. Worldwide, it is the fourth leading cause of disability, with projections for 2020 predicting it will become the second most disabling condition worldwide.[9] The disability is due to: (1) the high prevalence of depression; (2) a typically chronic or recurrent course; (3) the magnitude of the reduction in daily function directly attributable to the depressive syndrome; and (4) the life-shortening effects due directly to the disorder (e.g. through suicide) or indirectly due to increased mortality when depression co-occurs with GMCs (e.g. myocardial infarction).

Risk factors for developing a major depressive episode include gender, family history of depression, prior major depressive episodes and the presence of a GMC. The average age at the onset of MDD (i.e. the age of the first episode) is in the mid- to late twenties, though increasing rates of MDD have been found in those more recently born. Substantial numbers of adolescents suffer MDD. Women are twice as likely as men, especially during the reproductive years, to suffer MDD.[10]

MDD patients are divided into those with a single episode and those with recurrent episodes. The course of illness is marked by episodes lasting 6–18 months in most cases, but more long-lasting episodes are not uncommon. The time between episodes may be months to years. The greater the number of prior episodes, the more likely is the next episode.[11] A single episode is associated with a 50–80% risk of a second episode.[12,13] Two episodes beget a third episode in 70% of patients. There is a > 90% chance of a fourth episode for those with three prior episodes.[14]

Figure 5.2 provides exemplar courses of illness. In some instances, there is complete spontaneous recovery to an asymptomatic state (A), while many others (B) move into and out of MDEs, while continuing depressive symptoms characterize the interepisode periods. Most disabling are the even more chronic forms of the illness (C and D). In classic chronic MDD, the episode lasts > 2 years (C). In so-called 'double depression' (D), the illness begins with dysthymic disorder, but over time MDEs are superimposed on top of the continuing dysthymic disorder.

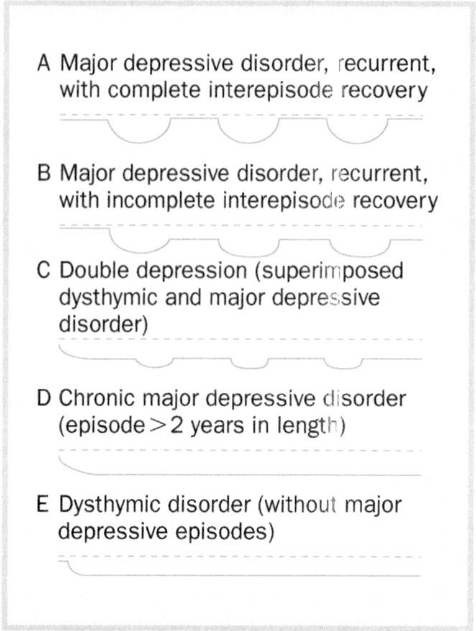

Most studies of clinical populations suggest that chronic depression (C) accounts for 5–15% of patients seen in psychiatric practice, while another 20–30% have double depression (D). Episodic depression with incomplete interepisode recovery (B) may account for another 30–50% of depressed patients seen by psychiatrists. Thus, the classic episodic course (A) represents the minority of clinical depressions in psychiatric care.[4]

Classic melancholic features such as anhedonia, unreactive mood, weight and

A Major depressive disorder, recurrent, with complete interepisode recovery

B Major depressive disorder, recurrent, with incomplete interepisode recovery

C Double depression (superimposed dysthymic and major depressive disorder)

D Chronic major depressive disorder (episode > 2 years in length)

E Dysthymic disorder (without major depressive episodes)

Figure 5.2
Exemplar courses of unipolar depressive illness. (Adapted, with permission, from Rush and Thase.[25])

appetite loss, profound guilt, early morning awakening, significant psychomotor slowing or agitation, and diurnal variation (with symptoms worse in the morning) are common in severe depression. Others (perhaps 20–30%) will report oversleeping (hypersomnia), weight/appetite gain, and have a reactive mood with exquisite sensitivity to perceived rejection by others (e.g. atypical symptom features). Of those with MDD, about 10–20% will suffer psychotic symptoms (e.g. hallucinations, delusions) when depressed.[4]

Bipolar disorder

Bipolar disorder is characterized by multiple MDEs (average 12/lifetime) interspersed with one or more hypomanic, but no manic, episodes (bipolar I disorder), or one or more manic episodes (bipolar II disorder). Manic episodes, typically lasting weeks to a few months, are very disabling, whereas hypomanic episodes (less than manic) are often seen as times of extreme productivity.[15]

So-called mixed episodes (episodes with both depressive and manic symptoms) may occur in 30–50% of patients with bipolar disorder. Common co-morbidities in bipolar I and II disorders include substance or alcohol abuse or dependence, and various anxiety disorders. Psychotic symptoms occur in about half of the major depressive and manic episodes seen in bipolar I disorder.

While classically viewed as episodic illnesses characterized by spontaneous, complete recovery between mood episodes (i.e. hypomanic, manic, depressive or mixed episodes), bipolar disorders often have significant, disabling mood symptoms between the full-blown mood episodes.

Both bipolar I and II disorders are viewed as lifelong, typically genetic, conditions that require lifelong treatment. However, some bipolar I or II syndromes may be caused by traumatic injury to the brain, neurological disorders (e.g. multiple sclerosis, stroke), medications (e.g. corticosteroids), or other

GMCs (e.g. hyperparathyroidism). Bipolar I disorder affects 0.8–1.2% of the population; bipolar II disorder affects 0.5–0.8% of the population. Each type of bipolar disorder tends to run in families, though relatives of those with bipolar I disorder may suffer bipolar II disorder and vice versa.[15]

Risk factors for bipolar disorder include a positive family history of bipolar I or II disorder, but gender is not a risk factor. Bipolar disorder is often a lethal condition due to the high rate of suicide, especially among those with concomitant substance abuse.

Chronic or recurrent courses of illness

As noted above, substantial numbers of persons with MDD, and virtually all persons with bipolar I or II disorder, have a recurrent or chronic course of illness. Importantly, many of these 'recurrent' illnesses are characterized by continuing symptoms in the periods between full-blown episodes that meet formal diagnostic criteria. Risk factors for recurrence/chronicity are listed in Box 5.1.[16] In recognition of the high prevalence of longer term, chronic, or recurrent courses of illness, most management guidelines now clearly recognize the need for longer term, effective, and well-tolerated treatments.[17,18]

Box 5.1
Risk factors for recurrence/chronicity.

- *Number of previous episodes[55]*
- *Number of days spent depressed during lifetime[56]*
- *Family history of major depressive disorder[57-59]*
- *History of key clinical variables, especially early age at onset[60]*
- *Chronic dysthymia[61]*
- *Psychosis[34]*
- *Treatment resistance[34]*
- *Prompt relapse or recurrence following previous discontinuation of treatment[62,63]*
- *Previous suicidal behavior or persistent suicidal ideation during depressive episodes[64]*
- *Presence of recurrences accompanied by one or more selected laboratory variables, notably: (1) persistent abnormalities of stress hormone regulation with elevated glucocorticoids or abnormal hypothalamic–pituitary–adrenal measures; (2) magnetic resonance imaging evidence of hippocampal or amygdala atrophy not attributable to other causes; or (3) selected sleep EEG abnormalities[65-68]*
- *Current severity; concurrent medical illness, or personal or occupational circumstances that make any future depressive recurrence truly 'hazardous'[69,70]*

Adapted from Greden.[16]

Overview of treatment options and issues

Phases of treatment

Treatment of MDD is classically divided into three phases: acute, continuation and maintenance (Figure 5.3). For bipolar disorder, similar phases apply, though virtually all patients require maintenance treatment.

Acute treatment aims at complete symptom removal and restoration of function. The reason to emphasize complete remission and not just improvement (after which clinically significant symptoms can remain) is that remitted, as opposed to improved but not fully remitted, depressive episodes are characterized by better daily function[19] and by a better prognosis.[20,21]

Acute phase treatment options may include medications, psychotherapy, the combination of both, or somatic treatments, such as electroconclusive therapy (ECT), VNS (where available) or light therapy. Often, a trial and error approach is used to determine which treatment(s), used singly or in combination, produce maximal symptom relief with minimal side-effect burden.

There is little evidence to guide the selection of the initial agents. Medications are generally of

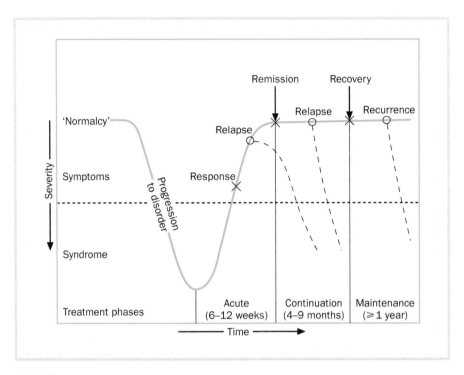

Figure 5.3
Phases of treatment. (Adapted, with permission, from the Depression Guideline Panel.[17])

equal efficacy, with a 50–60% response rate (and a 35–40% remission rate) expected after an 8-week trial (intent-to-treat sample) of MDD not characterized either by treatment resistance, chronicity, or complex co-morbidities (i.e. multiple concomitant psychiatric (Axis II) or general medical (Axis III) disorders). Some pooled analyses suggest greater efficacy for 'dual-action' agents (e.g. venlafaxine),[22] while other meta-analyses do not.[23]

Medication selection includes classic and newer antidepressants, such as bupropion, maprotiline, mianserin, mirtazapine, nefazodone, venlafaxine, monoamine oxidase inhibitors (MAOI), selective serotonin reuptake inhibitors (SSRI): citalopram, fluoxetine, fluvoxamine, paroxetine, or sertraline), and tricyclic agents. Short- and longer term side-effect burden and tolerability, potential drug–drug interactions, and other pharmacodynamic and pharmacokinetic features play a role in selecting available antidepressants. More recently, selected anticonvulsants have suggestive (open case series) or more definitive (i.e. controlled blinded trials) evidence of efficacy in depressions of the unipolar or bipolar type. For example, lamotrigine exceeded placebo in a large controlled trial of patients in the depressed phase of bipolar disorder.[24] However, those anticonvulsants with efficacy in mood disorders are more likely to have antimanic than antidepressant effects (e.g. divalproex, carbamazepine).

The major causes of failure of acute treatment are adherence, side-effect burden, inadequate dose, or inadequate duration of the initial treatment trial. Medication, or even depression-targeted, time-limited therapy, trials require 6–8 weeks to determine whether efficacy will follow. Longer treatment often is needed to determine if remission will result.

Few controlled studies guide the selection of the next treatment if the first treatment proves insufficiently effective or cannot be tolerated.[25,26] Treatment algorithms have been proposed,[27] but they are based substantially on open trials or small case series. Some studies indicate that a change in the medication class after the initial medication fails is effective in about 50% of non-responders to the first medication, whereas other open, uncontrolled trials support the notion of switching within the medication class of SSRI, again with a roughly 50% response rate to the second SSRI if the first SSRI is not well tolerated or is ineffective.[28]

Continuation phase treatment begins once the acute phase ends and aims at preventing the return of the most recent episode (a relapse). The continuation phase lasts 4–9 months (or longer) depending on how long the index episode would have continued spontaneously. Usually the same medication at the same dose as that used in the acute phase is recommended. Obviously, for more chronic courses of illness, when continuation ends and maintenance begins is nearly impossible to gauge.

Maintenance treatment aims at preventing a new episode of depression (a recurrence). Maintenance phase treatment is called for in both bipolar disorders and in highly recurrent or chronic forms of MDD. Various guidelines[17,18,27–30] recommend maintenance medication for MDD with three or more episodes and for MDD with two episodes (especially if closely spaced), and one or more risk factors for subsequent episodes (e.g. positive family history in a first-degree relative of recurrent MDD or bipolar disorder, incomplete recovery between the two episodes, onset of the first MDE before the age of 18, psychotic features in the first two episodes, etc.).

Maintenance treatment is typically conducted with the same doses and types of medications used to obtain remission (or at least a response) in the acute phase. A variety

Table 5.1
Double-blind, placebo-controlled discontinuation studies of antidepressant treatment in continuation and maintenance phases.

| Study | Relapse/Recurrence* | |
	Antidepressant (%)	Placebo (%)
Prien et al[71]	IMI (29)	85
Prien et al[71]	Li (41)	85
Coppen et al[72]	AMI (0)	31
Prien et al[71]	Li (57)	71
Schou[73]	Li (29)	84
Kane et al[74]	Li (29)	100
Kane et al[74]	IMI (67)	100 (NS)
Bjork[75]	ZIM (32)	84
Glen et al[76]	AMI (43)	88
Glen et al[76]	Li (42)	88
Prien et al[77]	IMI (44)	71
Montgomery et al[78]	FLU (26)	57
Georgotas et al[79]	PHN (13)	65
Frank et al[62]	IMI (21)	78
Rouillon et al[80]	MAP (16)	32
Jakovljevic and Mewett[81]	IMI (21)	78
Jakovljevic and Mewett[81]	PAR (14)	23 (NS)
Robinson et al[82]	PHN (10)	75
Doogan and Caillard[82]	SER (13)	46
Montgomery and Dunbar[84]	PAR (15)	39
Buysse et al[85]	NOR (27)	62
Bauer et al[86]†	Li (0)	47

AMI, Amitriptyline; FLU, fluoxetine; IMI, imipramine; Li, lithium; MAP, maprotyline; NOR, nortriptyline; PAR, paroxetine; PHN, phenelzine; SER, sertraline.
*All comparisons were significant (P < 0.05) except where shown as NS (non-significant).
†An augmenting trial.
Adapted from Greden.[16]

of placebo-controlled, double-blind discontinuation studies suggest the efficacy of medication (as opposed to placebo) in the continuation and maintenance phases of treatment (Table 5.1). Of note, however, are the 20–40% recurrence/relapse rates even under research conditions in these studies that exclude treatment-resistant recurrent depressions.

Issues in longer term treatment

Longer term/maintenance treatment is associated with a number of clinical challenges, including adherence, side-effect burden, and loss of effect, with the apparent need for changes in the medication regimen (i.e. changes in dose, in type of medication, or in both). Adherence is a problem in the care of all chronic medical conditions requiring long-term treatment. Adherence is exacerbated by side-effect burden, especially if additional medications must be added over time to sustain the benefit.

Most studies (Table 5.1) reveal that the long-term care of chronic/recurrent depressions is associated with loss of effect in 10–40% of patients over 1 year or so. Whether this 10–40% relapse/recurrence rate is due to non-adherence or loss of medication effect, even properly taken, is not well defined. The consequences of a loss of effect, however, are often changes in the dose, type and/or number of medications used. Thus, many patients with bipolar or unipolar disorders often end up on several psychotropic medications at the same time, with the apparent need to shuffle among medications over time to sustain the benefit initially obtained. Algorithms and guidelines for how to manage depressions that recur while being treated with maintenance phase medications do not exist. No randomized controlled trials (RCT) are available to recommend preferred practices for managing relapses/recurrences.

Treatment resistance

The topic of treatment resistance has only recently been emphasized in clinical research reports. Yet, from both a conceptual and clinical point of view, one can readily see that treatment resistance is extremely common in practice. Recall that only 35–45% of non-resistant major depressions remit with 8 weeks of treatment. Some additional depressions that respond by 10–12 weeks of acute treatment may remit over a subsequent 2–4 month time period.[27] Note that these numbers refer to populations that are not characterized by treatment resistance.

Since the aim of treatment is **sustained** remission (i.e. not just remission at the end of acute treatment), then whether those with remission at exit from acute treatment sustain that state over time must be examined. Koran et al[31] found that only 70% of those with chronic major depression who achieved symptomatic remission at acute treatment exit retained that status over the ensuing 4 months while on treatment. Of those with a response but without remission, about 40% did achieve remission, but a quarter to a third suffered relapses over the ensuing 4 months of continuation phase treatment.

While a chronic course does not automatically imply greater treatment resistance, the more chronic or recurrent disorders may be associated with a longer time to the onset of either response or remission.[32] Treatment resistance may vary along a continuum from moderately resistant (failure to achieve at least a response with one treatment) to very resistant (failure to achieve response with four or more different treatments). Various methods to 'stage' or rate resistance are available.[33] It is believed that a greater degree of resistance is associated with a lower probability of response to the next treatment.[34] This has been demonstrated with ECT using historical information to define the degree of resistance.[35–38] It is logical, but yet to be convincingly demonstrated prospectively, that greater degrees of medication resistance are associated with shorter periods of response or remission if the medication treatment is initially effective.

In sum, any depression for which a prolonged sustained remission cannot be obtained with a single, initial agent may be viewed as treatment resistant. If the first treatment leads to a 50% remission rate initially, and if 70% of these remitters maintain that status over the next year, then 65% of outpatients will have treatment-resistant depression (i.e. not achieve a sustained remission with the first treatment). If the second treatment leads to a 50% remission rate that is sustained in 70% of patients, then an additional 23% (i.e. 65% × 35%) will achieve sustained

remission. That leaves over 40% of patients needing yet another treatment trial, having not achieved a sustained remission with the first two treatments!

Given the substantial relapse/recurrence rates for patients continuing medication treatment over 6–12 months following the onset of at least a response, the need for a well-tolerated treatment that is associated with a sustained remission (preferably) or at least a sustained response is clear. From an economic perspective, the need is also clear. The cost of treatment-resistant depression has recently been estimated to be $40,000/year for those requiring one or more hospitalizations and $11,000/year for those able to be treated exclusively as outpatients, as compared to $6000/year for depressions that are not treatment resistant.[39]

Acute effects of vagus nerve stimulation (VNS) in clinical trials of depression

Given the well-justified need for an effective long-term treatment, an open-label, acute phase study was launched to describe the efficacy, safety, and tolerability of VNS when added to ongoing but stable medication regimens (or if used for patients on no treatment throughout the study). Subsequent to this open, 10-week acute trial, participants continued on VNS. During this naturalistic longer term follow-up phase, both VNS stimulation parameters and concomitant medication types or dosages could be modified based on clinical judgment. The study was conducted at the following institutions: (1) Baylor College of Medicine, Houston, Texas; (2) Columbia University College of Physicians and Surgeons and New York State Psychiatric Institute, New York, New York; (3) Medical University of South Carolina, Charleston, South Carolina; and (4) University of Texas Southwestern Medical Center, Dallas, Texas. Figure 5.4 summarizes the overall design of the study.

Participants

Men and women, 18–70 years of age, were eligible, except for pregnant women and those not using acceptable birth control methods.

Those with atypical or psychotic depressions and those with a history of schizophrenia, schizoaffective, or other non-mood psychotic disorders, and those with rapid cycling bipolar disorder (four or more mood episodes in the last year) were excluded. Also excluded were patients with clinically significant, current suicidal intent, and those with certain risks related to the surgical implantation and VNS stimulation. The average baseline 28-item Hamilton Rating Scale for Depression $(HRSD_{28})$[40,41] score had to be ≥ 20, and the Global Assessment of Function (GAF)[4] score had to be ≥ 50.

Patients had to be in a MDE as part of MDD, bipolar I, or bipolar II, disorder. The current MDE had to be 2 years in length, or there had to be more than four MDE in a lifetime. The current MDE had to have not

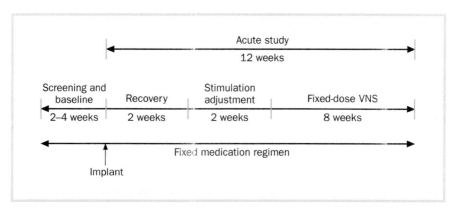

Figure 5.4
Overall design of the vagus nerve stimulation (VNS) study.

responded to at least two adequate antidepressant medication treatment trials with at least two different medication classes. Those with bipolar disorder had to be either resistant, intolerant, or have a medical contraindication to lithium. An adequate medication trial was defined by the Antidepressant Treatment History Form (ATHF).[42] Patients also must have had no substantial clinical improvement with psychotherapy of at least 6 weeks duration.

The ATHF gauged the degree of medication-resistance for the current MDE. The ATHF uses information obtained from patients, family members, treating physicians, medical records, and pharmacy logs. The ATHF rates each psychotropic medication trial on a 0–5 scale, with higher ratings denoting a longer trial at higher doses. An ATHF rating of ≥ 3 is required to define the trial as adequate. To illustrate, a score of 3 requires at least 4 weeks of fluoxetine at 20–39 mg/day or at least 4 weeks of imipramine at 200–299 mg/day. Categories of antidepressant treatments for MDD included heterocyclics/tricyclics, MAOI, SSRI, bupropion, mirtazapine, nefazodone, trazodone, venlafaxine, and ECT, while carbamazepine and lithium were also counted for bipolar disorder.

VNS treatment

The device implantation and treatment delivery were based on studies of VNS in treatment-resistant epilepsy.[43–46] After a 2–4 week baseline period, during which two measures of depressive symptom severity were obtained, the VNS generator was implanted and connected to the left vagus nerve using procedures identical to those used in epilepsy.[46]

Following implantation, patients were told that the device might or might not be activated (it was not activated in any patient) during a 2-week recovery period. Thereafter, the VNS dose was adjusted over a 2-week period – typically by increasing the amount of current to a tolerable level. For the next 8 weeks, VNS stimulation parameters were unchanged. Medication doses and types were unchanged from baseline through to the end of 10 weeks of VNS. In nearly all cases, stimulation parameters were 20 Hz, 0.5–1.5 mA, a duty cycle of 30 seconds on and 5 minutes off, and a 500 microsecond pulse width. Most dose adjustments entailed increases in the output current in 0.25 mA increments until a still tolerable level was reached over the 2-week VNS dose-adjustment period.

Concomitant therapy

Patients could receive antidepressant, mood stabilizer, or other psychotropic medications (e.g. atypical antipsychotics), as long as the same medication types and doses were constant from the baseline period through the 12 weeks following implantation.

Assessments

Efficacy and safety data were gathered at the two baseline (pre-implantation) visits, at weeks 1 and 2 following implantation, and at weeks 3 and 4 (the VNS adjustment period). Data in the fixed VNS dose period were obtained at weeks 5, 6, 8, 10, and 12 following implantation. The $HRSD_{28}$ and the 10-item Montgomery–Åsberg Depression Rating Scale (MADRS)[47] were used to measure depressive symptoms. Manic/hypomanic symptoms were rated by the Young Mania Rating Scale (YMRS).[48] Global severity and change measures included the Clinical Global Impressions– Improvement (CGI–I) and – Severity Index (CGI–SI),[49] while functional status was measured by the GAF and the Medical Outcomes Study Short Form – 36 (MOS SF–36).[50]

Sample characteristics

Table 5.2 shows that this 60-patient sample was characterized by high levels of depressive symptom severity, functional impairment, and longstanding illness (median duration of the current MDE was 6.6 years). Most (83%) had recurrent depressive episodes.

Table 5.3 summarizes the antidepressant treatment history for the current MDE. Nearly 16 different treatments (almost nine with traditional antidepressant medications) were tried in the current MDE. The strict scoring using the ATHF indicated that, on average, patients had not responded satisfactorily to nearly five adequate antidepressant trials during the current episode. Most (66.7%) patients had received ECT in their lifetime, of which 85% had received ECT during the current MDE. These multiple unsuccessful treatment attempts document the highly treatment-resistant nature of the sample.

Outcomes

Table 5.4 shows mean scores for each key outcome, with overall statistically significant improvements (all $P < 0.0001$) in $HRSD_{28}$, MADRS, GAF and CGI severity scores from baseline to acute study exit. Of the 59 patients, 18 (30.5%) evidenced a response (i.e. $\geq 50\%$ reduction in $HRSD_{28}$ scores). Of these 18 patients who received VNS, nine (15.3% of the initial sample) achieved a complete response (i.e. acute exit $HRSD_{28} \leq 10$). Of the 59 patients, 37.3% (22 of 59) received a CGI–I score of 1 or 2 (i.e. much or very much improved); only three patients were rated as minimally worse. There was no significant change in YMRS scores from baseline to acute study exit.

Table 5.2
Demographic and clinical characteristics of the sample (n = 60).

Characteristic	
Age at implant (years) (mean)	47
Female (%)	65
Caucasian (%)	98
Hispanic (%)	2
Unipolar MDD, recurrent (%)	47
Unipolar MDD, single episode (%)	27
Bipolar I or II disorder (%)	27
Baseline HRSD$_{28}$ total score (mean)	37
Baseline GAF total score (mean)	41
Median length of current episode (years)	7
Age at onset of current episode (years) (mean)	37
Total length of mood disorder (years) (mean)	18
Age at onset of mood disorder (years) (mean)	29

GAF, Global Assessment of Function; HRSD$_{28}$, Hamilton Rating Scale for Depression; MDD, major depressive disorder.
Adapted from Sackeim et al.[2]

Table 5.3
Medication treatments during the current major depressive episode (MDE) (n = 60).

	Mean	Range
Total medications	16	3–44
Antidepressants	9	1–21
Other mood disorder medications	5	0–16
Antidepressant Treatment History Form adequacy ratings		
Unsuccessful individual medication trials	5	2–14
Unsuccessful trials of categories of medication	4	2–9

Adapted from Sackeim et al.[2]

Table 5.4
Major outcomes at baseline (n = 60) and acute study exit (n = 59).

Rating scale	Baseline period* (mean)	Study exit (mean)	Change in baseline to exit (%) (mean)†
HRSD$_{28}$	37	25	32‡
MADRS	33	23	30†
CGI–I§	NA$^{\parallel}$	37	NA$^{\parallel}$
CGI–SI	5	4	23‡
GAF	41	57	44‡
YMRS	2	2	−12

CGI–I, CGI–SI, Clinical Global Impressions – Improvement and – Severity Index, respectively; GAF, Global Assessment of Function; HRSD$_{28}$, Hamilton Rating Scale for Depression; MADRS, Montgomery–Åsberg Repression Rating Scale; YMRS, Young Mania Rating Scale.
*Average of visits 1 and 2.
†Paired t-test on change scores.
‡P < 0.0001.
§CGI–I reported as the percentage of patients with a score of 1 or 2.
$^{\parallel}$Not applicable.
Adapted from Sackeim et al.[2]

Time course for symptom change

Figure 5.5 shows the average HRSD$_{28}$ score for subgroups classified as HRSD$_{28}$ responders or non-responders at the time of acute study exit (i.e. after 10 weeks of VNS). For responders, clinical improvement was gradual. Two-thirds of the 18 responders evidenced first response at or following 6 weeks of VNS (median time to first response was 45.5 days for responders).

Functional benefit

Table 5.5 summarizes selected MOS SF–36 subscores at baseline and acute study exit.

Marked baseline impairment is evident on multiple subscales relative to norms for both healthy and depressed individuals.[50] Responders, defined by the HRSD$_{28}$ at study exit, showed significant improvement in the mental component and on all subscales except for physical function and pain index (all P < 0.05). Interestingly, HRSD$_{28}$ non-responders at study exit also evidenced statistically significant, but smaller, improvements in the mental component, vitality, social function, and mental health subscales (all P < 0.05).

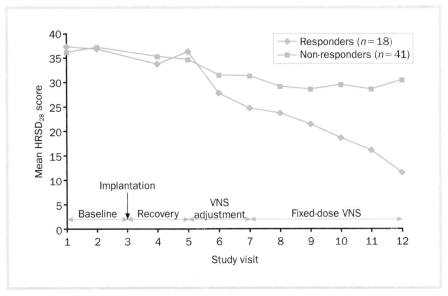

Figure 5.5
Mean Hamilton Rating Scale for Depression (HRSD$_{28}$) scores for responders (n = 18) and non-responders (n = 41) defined by acute study exit HRSD$_{28}$. Response defined as a ≥50% reduction in baseline HRSD$_{28}$ total score by acute study exit. VNS, Vagus nerve stimulation. (Adapted, with permission, from Sackeim et al.[2])

Safety and tolerability

No patient discontinued the acute study due to adverse events (AEs). Table 5.6 lists the types and incidences of AEs that may have been related to surgery and/or VNS stimulation occurring in ≥ 5% of patients. Holter monitoring data obtained over at least 12 hours collected at baseline (between visits 1 and 2) and at acute study exit (12 weeks post-implantation) (first 30 patients) revealed no significant changes.

Effects of VNS on neurocognitive function

Sackeim et al[51] reported on results of 13 neurocognitive tests obtained on 27 of the first 30 subjects included in the open trial of 59 patients noted above. No deterioration in any neurocognitive measure was found. In fact, improvements relative to baseline in executive functions (logical reasoning, working memory, response inhibition and impulsiveness), motor speed (finger tapping),

Table 5.5
Mean scores on the Medical Outcomes Study Short Form – 36 (MOS SF–36) for the Hamilton Rating Scale for Repression (HRSD$_{28}$) responders and non-responders at acute study exit.

	Responders (n = 17)		Non-responders (n = 41)	
	Baseline	Exit	Baseline	Exit
Mental component*	17	39†	17	21†
Physical component*	46	45	51	47
Subscales*				
Physical function	60	66	66	63
Role function	34	60†	57	47
Pain index	59	61	64	54
Health perceptions	49	62†	57	55
Vitality improvements	9	41†	12	18†
Social function	23	58†	22	27†
Role emotional	4	41†	13	10
Mental health	22	62†	22	27†

*Some patients did not complete all of the MOS SF–36 subscales.
†Statistically significant percentage improvement from baseline by paired t-test (P < 0.05).
Adapted from Sackeim et al.[2]

psychomotor function (digit symbol test), and language (verbal fluency) were found. For most measures, improved neurocognitive performance was related to the extent of reduction in depressive symptoms, but not to VNS current.

Predictors of clinical outcome

Univariate logistic regression analyses were used to identify factors that might predict VNS response (⩾ 50% reduction in HRSD$_{28}$ scores). Those not responding to larger numbers of adequate antidepressant treatment trials in the current MDE and those who received ECT in their lifetime and/or who did not respond well to ECT were less likely to respond to VNS. Patients without exposure to ECT were 3.9 times more likely to respond to VNS.

Multivariate analyses revealed that the number of unsuccessful adequate antidepressant treatment trials as defined by the ATHF during the index episode was highly related to VNS outcome (Figure 5.6). None of the 13 patients who had not responded to more than seven adequate antidepressant trials responded to 10 weeks of

Table 5.6
Percentage of patients reporting adverse events (possibly, probably, or definitely related to implantation or to stimulation).*

Adverse event	No. patients (%)	Adverse event	No. patients (%)
Voice alteration	55	Wound abnormality	7
Incision site pain	30	Nausea	7
Headache	22	Paresthesia	7
Neck pain	17	Rash	7
Coughing	17	Infection	5
Dyspnea	15	Tooth disorder	5
Pain	13	Dizziness	5
Dysphagia	13	Twitching	5
Pharyngitis	13	Insomnia	5
Dyspepsia	10	Palpitation	5

*For adverse events occurring in ≥5% of patients.
Adapted from Sackeim et al.[2]

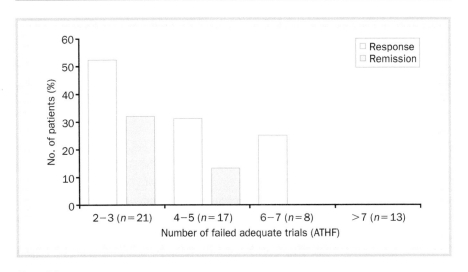

Figure 5.6
Response and remission rates [based on Hamilton Rating Scale for Depression (HRSD$_{28}$) score criteria] in relation to the number of failed adequate antidepressant treatment trials defined by the Antidepressant Treatment History Form (ATHF) during the current major depressive episode (n = 59). One placebo responder excluded. Response includes response with or without remission. (Adapted, with permission, from Sackeim et al.[2])

VNS, while the response rate (39.1%) was substantial among patients with less profound degrees of treatment resistance ($P = 0.0057$). It appears that response to 10 weeks of VNS is more likely for those with substantial, but not extreme, levels of treatment resistance. However, whether better outcomes may be found with longer term VNS, even in those with greater degrees of treatment resistance, remains to be determined.

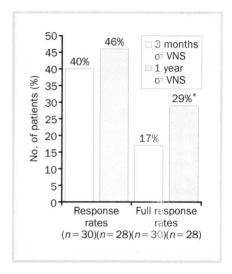

Figure 5.7
*Response [≥50% reduction in baseline Hamilton Rating Scale for Depression (HRSD$_{28}$) total score] and full response (HRSD$_{28}$ total score ≤10) rates after 3 months (acute study exit) and 1 year of vagus nerve stimulation (VNS). *McNemar's Exact Test (P = 0.046) comparing 3 months to 1 year of VNS. (Adapted, with permission, from Marangell et al.[3])*

Long-term effects of vagus nerve stimulation (VNS) in depression

Results obtained for longer term outcomes in the first 30 participants given VNS have recently been published.[3] In this group, 12 (40%) had a response to acute VNS. Within this group of 12, five (17% of the original 30 patients) achieved full responses (HRSD$_{28}$ ≤ 10). After an additional 9 months of VNS (during which both VNS stimulation parameters and/or medication types or doses could be changed based on clinical judgment), 46% were responders (with or without full response) and 29% were full responders (HRSD$_{28}$ ≤ 10). Response rates were unchanged, but the proportion of full responders increased ($P = 0.045$). Figure 5.7 shows these cross-sectional data.

Table 5.7 reveals that much of the benefit after 1 year of VNS was achieved with 6 months of VNS. Additional analyses revealed that those who benefited originally (i.e. after 10 weeks of VNS) largely retained the benefit at 12 months of VNS.

More recently, longer term 2-year follow-up data have been presented.[52–54] Results indicated that improvement in depressive symptoms measured by the HRSD$_{28}$ at study exit were sustained in HRSD$_{28}$ responders defined at exit from the 10-week acute VNS study. Importantly, in HRSD$_{28}$ acute study non-responders (i.e. those with <50%

Table 5.7
Clinical outcomes (observed cases).

Rating	Baseline (n = 30)	Acute exit (n = 30)	6 months (n = 29)	9 months (n = 27)	12 months (n = 28)
$HRSD_{28}$	38	23	19	19	20
MADRS	34	20	16	15	17
GAF	41	62	66	65	63
Response ($HRSD_{28}$) (%)*	NA†	40	55	52	46
Response (MADRS) (%)	NA†	30	62	52	50
Remission ($HRSD_{28}$ ≤10) (%)	NA†	17	31	33	29

GAF, Global Assessment of Function; HRSD, Hamilton Rating Scale for Depression; MADRS, Montgomery–Åsberg DepressionRating Scale.
*Response defined as a ≥50% reduction from baseline in $HRSD_{28}$ total score.
†Not applicable.
Adapted from Marangell et al.[3]

reduction in pretreatment $HRSD_{28}$ by exit from the 10-week acute study), significant reduction in $HRSD_{28}$ scores (26% reduction) was found at 2 years. As shown in Figure 5.8, the degree of treatment resistance was related to response and remission rates after a total of 1 year of VNS.[3]

Issues in selecting vagus nerve stimulation (VNS)

To date, evidence for the efficacy of acute and longer term VNS rests exclusively on open, uncontrolled trial data, which indicate a clinically significant rate of response (31%) and remission (15%) when VNS is added to ongoing but stable pharmacotherapy for 10 weeks.[2] It seems especially effective in the

moderately to severely treatment-resistant patients, but minimally effective (when delivered for 10 weeks) for the extremely treatment resistant. In the longer term, continuing VNS (along with pharmacotherapy) appears to be associated with sustained or growing benefits.[3] Evidence suggests increased remission rates over the longer term (1 year) and some reduction in depressive symptom severity even in acute study non-responders.[52–54] However, these longer term data were naturalistic and uncontrolled (meaning that both medication types and doses, as well as VNS stimulation parameters, could be changed in these longer term studies). Thus, one cannot conclusively attribute cause to VNS of these promising longer term outcomes. On the other hand, the

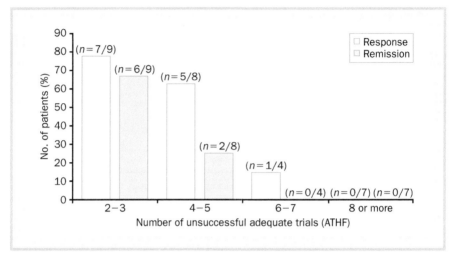

Figure 5.8
One year response and remission rates in relation to the number of unsuccessful treatment trials defined by the Antidepressant Treatment History Form (ATHF) during the current major depressive episode (n = 28). Two patients missed assessment. (Adapted, with permission, from Marangell et al.[3])

longstanding, chronic, recurrent, and treatment-resistant nature of the study sample is such that prolonged periods of sustained benefits would seem to be very unlikely given what is believed about the natural course of these disorders.

VNS is not available as a Food and Drug Administration (FDA)-approved treatment for depression in the United States, although it is available in Europe and Canada. Where might this intervention seem to fit in the overall treatment plan for such conditions? It would seem that several conditions apply to the consideration of VNS: (1) the prior course of

illness must indicate the need for a long-term treatment; (2) reasonable trials of several medications and at least one depression-targeted course of psychotherapy should have failed to result in sustained remission; (3) the continuing level of depressive symptoms and the associated impairment of daily function must be significant enough to warrant additional treatment; (4) preferably, the prior course of treatments should not indicate an extreme degree of treatment resistance (i.e. failure of seven or more different medication classes given at an adequate dose for an adequate duration); and (5) the patient and family must be willing to consent to VNS. It would seem reasonable to consider VNS as an option (where it is available) following two to four medication monotherapy attempts and at least one evidence-based augmentation effort (e.g. lithium plus a tricyclic).

Patients and clinicians will differ regarding what a sufficient number of adequate medication trials needs to be before considering VNS. For some patients, the convenience of VNS and its very modest long-term side-effect burden will make it more appealing earlier in a sequence of treatment attempts. For others, more medication trials may be desired before considering an intervention that entails surgery. Importantly, there is substantial evidence of the longer-term safety and tolerability of VNS in patients with epilepsy or depression. The decision to recommend VNS for the treatment of depression, based on currently available data, remains an individual patient and clinician choice.

Future directions

Clearly, additional data are needed to further establish both the indicators for and the overall efficacy of VNS for chronic and recurrent depressions with various degrees of treatment resistance. Such studies might entail additional acute phase RCT, blinded, controlled discontinuation trials of VNS in patients for whom it appears to be acutely

effective, longer term comparative trials of VNS versus medication algorithms, or other trial designs. In addition to acute and longer term efficacy studies, further attempts to identify baseline predictors of longer term non-response, whether some types of medications are particularly helpful when combined with VNS, and studies to identify optimal stimulation parameters for VNS will be needed. Finally, the longer term effects of VNS on the considerable economic and personal costs of chronic or recurrent depression deserve study.

References

1. Rush AJ, George MS, Sackeim HS et al. Vagus nerve stimulation (VNS) for treatment-resistant depressions: a multicenter study. Biol Psychiatry 2000; 47:276–86.

2. Sackheim HA, Rush AJ, George MS et al. Vagus nerve stimulation (VNS™) for treatment-resistant depression: efficacy, side effects, and predictors of outcome. Neuropsychopharmacology 2001; 25:713–28.

3. Marangell LB, Rush AJ, George MS et al. Vagus nerve stimulation (VNS) for major depressive episodes: one year outcomes. Biol Psychiatry 2002; 51:280–7.

4. American Psychiatric Association. Diagnostic and Statistical Manual of Mental Disorders, 4th edn. (American Psychiatric Association, Washington, DC, 1994.)

5. Bush DE, Ziegelstin RC, Tayback M et al. Even minimal symptoms of depression increase mortality risk after acute myocardial infarction. Am J Cardiol 2001; 88:337–41.

6. Lésperance F, Frasure-Smith N, Talajic M, Bourassa MG. Five-year risk of cardiac mortality in relation to initial severity and one-year changes in depression symptoms after myocardial infarction. Circulation 2002; 105:1049–53.

7. Gillen R, Tennen H, McKee TE et al. Depressive symptoms and history of depression predict rehabilitation efficiency in stroke patients. Arch Phys Med Rehabil 2001; 82:1645–9.

8. Egede LE, Zheng D, Simpson K. Comorbid depression is associated with increased health care use and expenditures in individuals with diabetes. Diabetes Care 2002; 25:464–70.

9. Murray CJ, Lopez AD. Alternative projections of mortality and disability by cause 1990–2020: Global Burden of Disease Study. Lancet 1997; 349:1498–504.

10. Rush AJ, Stewart RS, Garver DL, Waller DA. Neurological bases for psychiatric disorders. In: (Rosenberg RN, Pleasure DE, eds) Comprehensive Neurology, 2nd edn. (Raven Press, New York, 1998) 887–919.

11. Angst J. Major depression in 1998: are we providing optimal therapy? J Clin Psychiatry 1999; 60(Suppl 6):5–9.

12. Andrews G. Should depression be managed as a chronic disease? BMJ 2001; 322:419–21.

13. Mueller TI, Leon AC, Keller MB. Recurrence after recovery from major depressive disorder during 15 years of observational follow-up. Am J Psychiatry 1999; 156:1000–6.

14. Depression Guideline Panel. Clinical Practice Guideline. Number 5. Depression in Primary Care: Volume 1. Detection and Diagnosis. (US Dept of Health and Human Services, Agency for Health Care Policy and Research, Rockville, MD, 1993) AHCPR publication No. 93-0550.

15. Goodwin FK, Jamison KR. Manic-Depressive Illness. (Oxford University Press, New York, 1990.)

16. Greden JF (ed). Treatment of Recurrent Depression. Review of Psychiatry, Volume 20, Number 5. (American Psychiatric Publishing, Inc.: Washington, DC, 2002.)

17. Depression Guideline Panel. Clinical Practice Guideline. Number 5. Depression in Primary Care: Volume 2. Treatment of Major Depression. (US Dept of Health and Human Services, Agency for Health Care Policy and Research, Rockville, MD, 1993) AHCPR Publication No. 93-0551.

18. American Psychiatric Association. Practice guideline for the treatment of patients with major depressive disorder (revision). Am J Psychiatry 2000; 157(Suppl 4):1–45.

19. Miller IW, Keitner GI, Schatzerg AF et al. The treatment of chronic depression, Part 3: Psychosocial functioning before and after treatment with sertraline or imipramine. J Clin Psychiatry 1998; 59:608–19.

20. Judd LL, Akiskal HS, Maser JD et al. Major depressive disorder: a prospective study of residual subthreshold depressive symptoms as predictor of rapid relapse. J Affect Disord 1998; 50:97–108.

21. Judd LL, Paulus MJ, Schettler PJ et al. Does incomplete recovery from first lifetime major depressive episode herald a chronic course of illness? Am J Psychiatry 2000; 157:1501–4.

22. Thase ME, Entsuah AR, Rudolph RL. Remission rates during treatment with venlafaxine or selective serotonin reuptake inhibitors. Br J Psychiatry 2001; 178:234–41.

23. Freemantle N, Anderson IM, Young P. Predictive value of pharmacological activity for the relative efficacy of antidepressant drugs. Meta-regression analysis. Br J Psychiatry 2000; 177:292–302.

24. Calabrese JR, Bowden CL, Sachs GS et al. A double-blind placebo-controlled study of lamotrigine monotherapy in outpatients with bipolar I depression. Lamictal 602 Study Group. J Clin Psychiatry 1999; 60:79–88.

25. Rush AJ, Thase ME. Strategies and tactics in the treatment of chronic depression. J Clin Psychiatry 1997; 58(Suppl 13):14–22.

26. Thase ME, Rush AJ. When at first you don't succeed: sequential strategies for antidepressant nonresponders. J Clin Psychiatry 1997; 58(Suppl 13):23–9.

27. Crismon ML, Trivedi M, Pigott TA et al. The Texas Medication Algorithm Project. Report of the Texas Consensus Conference Panel on medication treatment of major depressive disorder. J Clin Psychiatry 1999; 60:142–56.

28. Bauer M, Whybrow PC, Angst J et al. World Federation of Societies of Biological Psychiatry (WFSBP) guidelines for biological treatment of unipolar depressive disorders, Part 2: Maintenance treatment of major depressive disorder and treatment of chronic depressive disorders and subthreshold depressions. World J Biol Psychiatry 2002; 3:67–84.

29. Rosenbaum JF, Fava M, Nierenberg AA, Sachs G. Treatment-resistant mood disorders. In: (Gabbard GO, ed.) Treatments of Psychiatric Disorders, Volume 2, 3rd edn. (American Psychiatric Publishing, Inc., Washington, DC, 2001) 1307–86.

30. Trivedi MH, DeBattista C, Fawcett J et al. Developing treatment algorithms for unipolar depression in cyberspace: International Psychopharmacology Algorithm Project (IPAP). Psychopharmacol Bull 1998; 34:355–9.

31. Koran LM, Gelenberg AJ, Kornstein SG et al.

Sertraline versus imipramine to prevent relapse in chronic depression. J Affect Disord 2001; 65:27–36.

32. Keller MB. Long-term treatment of recurrent and chronic depression. J Clin Psychiatry 2001; 62(Suppl 24):3–5.

33. Thase ME, Rush AJ. Treatment resistant depression. In: (Bloom FE, Kupfer DJ, eds) Psychopharmacology: The Fourth Generation of Progress. (Raven Press, New York, 1995) 1081–97.

34. Nierenberg AA, Amsterdam JD. Treatment-resistant depression: definition and treatment approaches. J Clin Psychiatry 1990; 51(Suppl 6):39–47.

35. Prudic J, Haskett RF, Mulsant F et al. Resistance to antidepressant medications and short-term clinical response to ECT. Am J Psychiatry 1996; 153:985–92.

36. Prudic J, Sackeim HA, Devanand DP. Medication resistance and clinical response to electroconvulsive therapy. Psychiatry Res 1990; 31:287–96.

37. Sackeim HA, Prudic J, Devanand DP et al. The impact of medication resistance and continuation pharmacotherapy on relapse following response to electroconvulsive therapy in major depression. J Clin Psychopharmacol 1990; 10:96–104.

38. Sackeim HA, Prudic J, Devanand DP et al. A prospective, randomized, double-blind comparison of bilateral and right unilateral electroconvulsive therapy at different stimulus intensities. Arch Gen Psychiatry 2000; 57:425–34.

39. Crown WH, Finkelstein S, Berndt ER et al. The impact of treatment-resistant depression on healthcare utilization and costs. J Clin Psychiatry (in press).

40. Hamilton M. A rating scale for depression. J Neurol Neurosurg Psychiatry 1960; 23:56–62.

41. Hamilton M. Development of a rating scale for primary depressive illness. Br J Soc Clin Psychol 1967; 6:278–96.

42. Sackeim HA. The definition and meaning of treatment-resistant depression. J Clin Psychiatry 2001; 62(Suppl 16):10–17.

43. Ben-Menachem E, Mañon-Espaillat R, Ristanovic R et al. Vagus nerve stimulation for treatment of partial seizures. 1. A controlled study of effect on seizures. First International Vagus Nerve Stimulation Study Group. Epilepsia 1994; 35:616–26.

44. The Vagus Nerve Stimulation Study Group. A randomized controlled trial of chronic vagus nerve stimulation for treatment of medically intractable seizures. Neurology 1995; 45:224–30.

45. Handforth A, DeGiorgio CM, Schachter SC et al. Vagus nerve stimulation therapy for partial-onset seizures: a randomized active-control trial. Neurology 1998; 51:48–55.

46. DeGiorgio CM, Amar A, Apuzzo MLJ. Surgical anatomy, implantation technique, and operative complications. In: (Schachter SC, Schmidt D, eds) Vagus Nerve Stimulation. (Martin Dunitz, Ltd, London, 2001) 31–50.

47. Montgomery SA, Åsberg M. A new depression scale designed to be sensitive to change. Br J Psychiatry 1979; 134:382–9.

48. Young RC, Biggs JT, Ziegler VE, Meyer DA. A rating scale for mania: reliability, validity and sensitivity. Br J Psychiatry 1978; 133:429–35.

49. Guy W. ECDEU Assessment Manual for Psychopharmacology. Revised Edition. (Superintendent of Documents, US Government Printing Office, US Department of Health, Education and Welfare, Washington, DC). DHEW Publication No. 76-338, 1976.

50. Ware JE, Sherbourne CD. The MOS 36-item short form health survey (SF-36). I. Conceptual framework and item selection. Med Care 1992; 30:473–83.

51. Sackeim HA, Keilp JG, Rush AJ et al. The effects of vagus nerve stimulation on cognitive performance in patients with treatment-resistant depression. Neuropsychiatr Neuropsychol Behav Neurol 2001; 14:53–62.

52. Marangell LB, George MS, Rush AJ et al. Vagus nerve stimulation (VNS) continues to show therapeutic benefit for chronic or recurrent treatment resistant depression up to two years after implant. US Psychiatric & Mental Health Congress, Boston, MA, November 15–18, 2001.

53. George MS, Rush AJ, Sackeim HA et al. Vagus nerve stimulation (VNS) continues to show therapeutic benefit for chronic or recurrent treatment resistant depression up to two years after implant. American College of Neuropsychopharmacology, Waikoloa, Hawaii, December 9–13, 2001.

54. Martinez JM, George MS, Rush AJ et al. Vagus nerve stimulation shows benefits in treatment-resistant depression for up to two years. American Psychiatric Association, Philadelphia, PA, May 18–23, 2002.

55. Greden JF. Antidepressant maintenance medications: when to discontinue and how to stop. J Clin Psychiatry 1993; 54:39–45.

56. Sheline YI, Sanghavi M, Mintun MA, Gado MH. Depression duration but not age predicts hippocampal volume loss in medically healthy women with recurrent

major depression. J Neurosci 1999; 19:5034–43.

57. Kendler KS, Kessler RC, Neale MC et al. The prediction of major depression in women: toward an integrated etiologic model. Am J Psychiatry 1993; 150:1139–48.

58. Kendler KS, Neale MC, Kessler RC et al. A longitudinal twin study of 1-year prevalence of major depression in women. Arch Gen Psychiatry 1993; 50:843–52.

59. Kendler KS, Karkowski LM, Prescott CA. Causal relationship between stressful life events and the onset of major depression. Am J Psychiatry 1999; 156:837–41.

60. Pine DS, Cohen P, Gurley D et al. The risk for early adulthood anxiety and depressive disorders in adolescents with anxiety and depressive disorders. Arch Gen Psychiatry 1998; 55:56–64.

61. Keller MB. The long-term treatment of depression. J Clin Psychiatry 1999; 60(Suppl 17):41–5.

62. Frank E, Kupfer DJ, Perel JM et al. Three-year outcomes for maintenance therapies in recurrent depression. Arch Gen Psychiatry 1990; 47:1093–9.

63. Kupfer DJ, Frank E, Perel JM et al. Five-year outcome for maintenance therapies in recurrent depression. Arch Gen Psychiatry 1992; 49:769–73.

64. Pfeffer C. The Suicidal Child. (Guildford Press, New York, 1986.)

65. Greden JF, Gardner R, King D et al. Dexamethasone suppression tests in antidepressant treatment of melancholia. The process of normalization and test-retest reproducibility. Arch Gen Psychiatry 1983; 40:493–500.

66. Sheline YI, Wang P, Gado M et al.

Hippocampal atrophy in recurrent major depression. Proc Natl Acad Sci USA 1996; 93:3908–13.

67. Kupfer DJ, Ehlers CL, Frank E et al. Persistent effects of antidepressants: EEG sleep studies in depressed patients during maintenance treatment. Biol Psychiatry 1994; 35:781–93.

68. Perlis M, Giles D, Buysse D et al. Self-reported sleep disturbance as a prodromal symptom in recurrent depression. J Affect Disord 1997; 42:209–12.

69. Cassem EH. Depressive disorders in the medically ill. An overview. Psychosomatics 1995; 36:S2–S10.

70. North CS, Ryall JE. Psychiatric illness in female physicians. Are high rates of depression an occupational hazard? Postgrad Med 1997; 101:233–6, 239–40, 242.

71. Prien RF, Klett J, Caffey EM Jr. Lithium carbonate and imipramine in prevention of affective episodes: A comparison in recurrent affective illness. Arch Gen Psychiatry 1973; 29:420–5.

72. Coppen A, Peet M, Bailey J et al. Double-blind and open prospective studies in lithium prophylaxis in affective disorders. Psychiatr Neurol Neurochir 1973; 76:500–10.

73. Schou M. Lithium research at the Psychopharmacology Research Unit, Risskov, Denmark. In: (Schou M, Stromgren E, eds) A Historical Account in Origin, Prevention and Treatment of Affective Disorders. (Academic Press, London, 1979) 1–8.

74. Kane JM, Quitkin FM, Rifkin A et al. Lithium carbonate and imipramine in the prophylaxis of unipolar and bipolar II illness: a prospective placebo-controlled comparison. Arch Gen Psychiatry 1982; 39:1065–9.

75. Bjork K. The efficacy of zimelidine in preventing depressive episodes in recurrent major depressive disorders – a double-blind placebo-controlled study. Acta Psychiatr Scand 1983; 308(Suppl):182–9.

76. Glen AIM, Johnson AL, Shepherd M. Continuation therapy with lithium and amitriptyline in unipolar depressive illness: a randomized double-blind controlled trial. Psychol Med 1984; 14:37–50.

77. Prien RF, Kupfer DJ, Mansky PA et al. Drug therapy in the prevention of recurrences in unipolar and bipolar affective disorders. Report of the NIMH Collaborative Study Group comparing lithium carbonate, imipramine, and a lithium carbonate–imipramine combination. Arch Gen Psychiatry 1984; 41:1096–104.

78. Montgomery SA, Dufour H, Brion S et al. The prophylactic efficacy of fluoxetine in unipolar depression. Br J Psychiatry 1988; 153(Suppl 3):69–76.

79. Georgotas A, McCue RE, Cooper TB. A placebo-controlled comparison of nortriptyline and phenelzine in maintenance therapy of elderly depressed patients. Arch Gen Psychiatry 1989; 46:783–6.

80. Rouillon F, Serrurier D, Miller H, Gerard MJ. Prophylactic efficacy of maprotiline on unipolar depression relapse. J Clin Psychiatry 1991; 52:423–31.

81. Jackovljevic M, Mewett S. Comparison between paroxetine, imipramine and placebo in preventing recurrent major depressive episodes. Eur Neuropsychopharmacol 1991; 1:440.

82. Robinson DS, Lerfald SC, Bennett B et al. Continuation and maintenance treatment of major depression with the monoamine oxidase inhibitor phenelzine: a double-blind placebo-controlled discontinuation study. Psychopharmacol Bull 1991; 27:31–9.

83. Doogan DP, Caillard V. Sertraline in the prevention of depression. Br J Psychiatry 1992; 160:217–22.

84. Montgomery SA, Dunbar GS. Paroxetine is better than placebo in relapse prevention and the prophylaxis of recurrent depression. Int Clin Psychopharmacol 1993; 8:189–95.

85. Buysse D, Reynolds C, Hoch C et al. Longitudinal effects of nortriptyline on EEG sleep and the likelihood of recurrence in elderly depressed patients. Neuropsychopharmacology 1996; 14:243–52.

86. Bauer M, Bschor T, Kunz D et al. Double-blind, placebo-controlled trial of the use of lithium to augment antidepressant medication in continuation treatment of unipolar major depression. Am J Psychiatry 2000; 157:1429–35.

Vagus nerve stimulation in the treatment of morbid obesity

Mitchell Roslin and Marina Kurian

6

Introduction

Obesity is defined as having excess adiposity or fat tissue. It is the result of caloric intake exceeding energy expenditure. As the body's most energy dense tissue, adipose tissue is the site where this excess energy is stored. Since it is more practical to measure height and weight, rather than the amount of fat, determination of the level of obesity is generated using these numbers. The most accurate numerical assessment is obtained by determining the body mass index (BMI). This number is derived by dividing weight (kilograms) by height (meters) squared. A BMI of > 40 is considered morbidly obese. As an example, an individual who is 5 feet 10 inches (about 1.78 m) tall and weighs 280 pounds (about 127 kg) has a body mass index of 40. A patient with a BMI of 25–30 is considered overweight, of 30–35 has stage I obesity, of 35–40 has stage II obesity and of > 40 has stage III or morbid obesity.

In the opinion of many health care experts, obesity is the largest health problem facing westernized societies. From a medical standpoint, obesity is the primary risk factor for type 2 diabetes and obstructive sleep apnea. It increases the chances for heart disease, pulmonary disease, infertility, osteoarthritis, cholecystitis and several major cancers, including breast and colon. From an economic standpoint, it is estimated that 100 billion dollars are spent on obesity and treating its major co-morbidities. This does not even consider the psychological and social costs of this epidemic problem.

Despite these alarming facts, treatment options for obesity remain limited. It is estimated that 50–60% of the population of the USA are obese or overweight. Of these patients, 5–6% are considered morbidly obese because they are approximately 100 pounds (about 45 kg) above their ideal body weight. Treatment options include dietary modification, very low calorie liquid diets, pharmaceutical agents, counseling, exercise programs and surgery. Surgical procedures that restrict the size of the stomach and/or bypass parts of the intestine are the only remedies that provide lasting weight loss for the majority of morbidly obese individuals. Surgical procedures for morbid obesity are becoming more common based on the long-term successful weight loss results.[1,2]

Increased awareness regarding the dangers of obesity, combined with the fact that these procedures are now being done with a laparoscope, in a minimally invasive manner, have made these procedures the fastest growing area of surgery in the United States. It is estimated that 80,000 operative procedures will be performed for obesity in 2002 in the USA. Vertical banded gastroplasty and gastric banding are restrictive procedures, and gastric bypass and biliopancreatic diversion (BPD) are restrictive/malabsorptive procedures. Even though done minimally invasively, these procedures are still major surgery, and have the potential for short-term complications and long-term nutritional problems. In some respects, surgery for obesity is forced behaviour modification; other less drastic options have not been successful in providing sustained weight loss. An optimal treatment for morbid obesity is not yet at hand.

The etiology of obesity is multifactorial. It is the combination of a genetic predisposition and environmental factors. But it is important to note that excess adiposity is the result of energy intake exceeding energy expenditure. Treatment has focused on reducing caloric intake and encouraging exercise to develop muscle and increase energy utilization. Presently, even surgical interventions are targeted at the gastrointestinal tract and limiting intake. Energy regulation is controlled by the central nervous system. Thus, it has been the present authors' contention that ideal long-term treatments would need to target the central nervous system and the gut–brain interaction.

Role of vagus nerve afferents in eating behavior

The termination of a meal or eating in humans is complex, and a full understanding of satiety and food consumption has remained elusive. It involves the interaction of cognitive factors from the cerebrum, feedback from the gastrointestinal tract as well as peripheral signals including messages from fat-storing adipocytes. Hormonal influences and peripheral and central monitors of blood glucose content are also involved. While there is feedback from all areas of the gastrointestinal tract to the brain, distension of the stomach is the single greatest factor in satiety. This has been shown by experiments that have placed a cuff around the pylorus. As a result, the stomach distends, activating mechanical receptors and the animal stops eating. Clinically, this accounts for the success of gastric stapling or banding in reducing food intake. What is most interesting as this happens is that there is an increase in vagus nerve activity.[3,4]

The vagus nerve is best known to physicians for its roles in acid production and motility. However, it is predominantly a sensory nerve and approximately 85% of its fibers are sensory or afferent. While there is a large overlap in the areas innervated by the right and left trunks, they are not mirror images. The anterior (left) vagus nerve provides the bulk of innervation to the proximal stomach. In contrast, the posterior trunk (right vagus nerve) provides the majority of the innervation to the pylorus and duodenum.

Evidence of the vagus nerve's role in eating behavior comes from multiple sources. As mentioned above, there is an increase in vagus nerve activity with gastric distension and food intake. More convincing are experiments that have been done with peptides known to reduce food intake in animal models: the most extensively studied is cholecystokinin (CCK). CCK is released after meal consumption. It is known to cause contraction of the gall bladder causing the release of bile to aid in fat digestion. Additionally, it helps control the release of chyme from the antrum of the stomach into the duodenum. The administration of CCK, either intravenously or into the peritoneum, has been shown to reduce food intake in animal models ranging from rodent to primate. These studies have been done with gastric fistulas to prevent distension and activation of mechanical receptors. Interestingly, surgical vagotomy attenuates this response. Furthermore, capsaicin, a chemical that damages or destroys vagal afferents, preserving efferents, also significantly reduces the effect of CCK. This data demonstrates that afferent vagus fibers are responsible for the satiating effect of CCK.[5,6] Recent research has indicated that the hepatic branch of the vagus is the area of action for CCK and the location of the bulk of CCK receptors. Several other peptides have also been studied with similar results. In fact, in a recent review, Bray[6] concluded that the vagus nerve is responsible for the transmission of the majority of afferent signals responsible for satiety.

In addition to peptides released and mechanical stretch, meal content is an important determinant of food intake. The administration of intravenous alimentation with fat and sugar has been shown to reduce food intake. Experiments have been performed in which a gastric fistula is created with fatty acids, simple sugars and amino acids being infused into the duodenum. Administration of oleic acid, a fatty acid, reduces food intake. Vagotomy and capsaicin markedly blunt this effect. Sugar infusion with maltose also reduces intake in a fistula model. While vagotomy blunts this effect, it is not nearly as dramatic as with fatty acids [6,7] This has led to the conclusion that lipoprivic feeding is controlled by vagally mediated peripheral signals. In comparison, glucoprivic feeding is controlled by the gastrointestinal tract and the central nervous system, and is only partially vagally mediated. A possible explanation is that glucose is the primary fuel of the central nervous system and as a result, it is therefore reasonable that the brain would preserve a role in monitoring adequate sugar intake.

Preclinical program

The combination of the anatomic relationship of the vagus nerve to the gastrointestinal tract, and the above physiologic experiments, provided the rationale for the investigation of electrical stimulation of the vagus nerve for

obesity and development of a preclinical animal experimental program. Despite this appealing theory, there was one major factor that needed to be considered prior to beginning investigation. During the numerous clinical years accumulated with vagus nerve stimulation for epilepsy, besides a few anecdotal reports, no weight loss was reported. Thus, several modifications were necessary. Since it was hoped to stimulate the small unmyelinated C fibers of the nerve, it was considered best to be in closer proximity to the gastroesophageal junction. Such positioning would avoid stimulation of fibers that join the trunk from the heart and lungs, and it was speculated that there was a greater likelihood of stimulating the target fibers. Additionally, positioning away from the neck and the recurrent laryngeal nerve would allow delivery of higher levels of current, which may be necessary to stimulate these unmyelinated fibers. Finally, since the right and left trunks have different distributions in the abdomen, and the contribution of both could be essential, it was decided to investigate bilateral stimulation of the vagus nerve.

To test whether vagus nerve stimulation (VNS) could alter food intake, a canine study was conducted. Ten mongrel dogs were divided into two different stimulation patterns: (1) acute studies, which were stimulated with duty cycles for 20 minutes before and during meal consumption; (2) chronic studies, which were stimulated with duty cycles continuously. Animals were fed twice daily and eating behavior, time of food consumption, and amount of food consumption was recorded.

A VNS Therapy bipolar lead was placed on each of the right and left vagal trunks via a left thoracotomy and attached to separate pulse generators. Animals were allowed 20 minutes to consume their meal: intake amount and time of consumption was observed and recorded. When the animal returned to baseline eating behavior and seemed sufficiently recovered from the surgical procedure (5–10 days), the VNS Therapy systems were activated. All animals were given unlimited access to water. All dogs were weighed on a weekly basis.

Output current (mA), duty cycle (on/off time), signal frequency (Hz) and pulse width (microseconds) was adjusted by placing the VNS Therapy Programming Wand Model 200 over the pulse generator on the skin.

No significant surgical complications were observed in any animal. One study was terminated on post-implant day 100 due to an erosion of one of the pulse generators through the skin. This was probably due to a combination of rapid loss of subcutaneous fat and placement of the pulse generator within the subcutaneous plane.

The studies were divided into two groups. Group I studies were performed using thoracic placement of the bipolar leads and acute stimulation parameters (stimulation

signals delivered 20 minutes before and during mealtime only). Group II studies consisted of eight animals, which had thoracic placement of the bipolar leads and chronic stimulation parameters (stimulation signals delivered at various duty cycles continuously throughout the day). As shown, during periods when the vagus nerve was stimulated (stimulation on), the average consumption time (time to consume a meal) increased from approximately 3.5 to 20 minutes. When the stimulation was turned off, the consumption time decreased from 20 minutes back down to approximately 3.5 minutes. The associated weight was also shown during this time (Figure 6.1). Analyses were performed on all studies in both groups, and included time of food consumption, amount of food consumed, change in weight, and hematologic and biochemical profiles.

Change in weight (weight at or closest to that at the time of NCP system implant minus weight at a specific time) was evaluated in the group I and II animals. Weight loss was observed in all chronically stimulated animals, except for one animal that was done early in the series. The percentage change in weight from the start of stimulation periods was calculated and compared in groups of days (Figure 6.2). A marked and statistically relevant change (decrease) in weight was observed in the chronically stimulated (group II) animals as compared to the animals undergoing acute stimulation (group I).

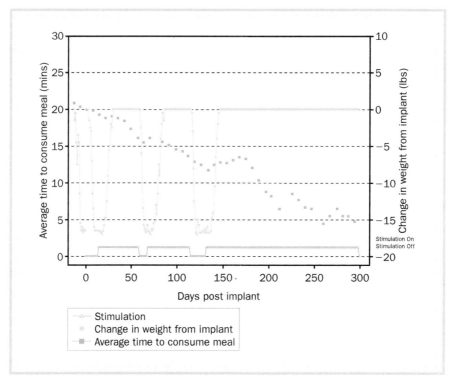

Figure 6.1
Chronic bilateral vagus nerve stimulation for the treatment of obesity. Animal # 1964. Time to consume meal and change in weight.

In summary, this study suggests that the use of bilateral VNS is effective in changing eating behavior, with a corresponding weight loss, in a canine animal model (Table 6.1). The poor response during acute VNS combined with the delayed effect of chronic stimulation suggests that VNS results in changes in the central nervous system and secondarily alters food intake.

Human pilot program

The combination of the results of the above study and the known safety of VNS in humans served as the basis for initiating a phase I study. A total of six patients underwent implantation of bilateral vagus nerve stimulators in the thoracic cavity at Lenox Hill Hospital, New York, and the

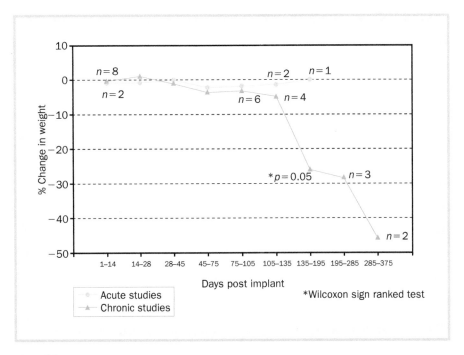

Figure 6.2
Vagus nerve stimulation for the treatment of obesity. Percentage change in weight from start of stimulation: chronic and acute study animals.

University of Texas, Houston. There were five females and a single male. All met clinical criteria for morbid obesity surgery. Following implantation, patients were blinded to the timing of activation of their generators: settings were a pulse width of 500 milliseconds, an on time of 30 seconds and an off time of 3 minutes, a frequency of 20 Hz, and amplitude starting at 0.25 mA (amplitude was raised to the maximum allowed by the generators over a several week period).

Results of this pilot study were mixed. One female, who was over 400 pounds (about 181 kg), lost > 90 pounds (about 41 kg) and continues to do well. Another lost 40 pounds (about 18 kg), became pregnant and had to leave the study. Two others lost approximately 10% of their body weight and then saturated. In the final two patients there was no effect.

While these early results compare favorably to current pharmaceutical options, they do not compare to the results that can be

Table 6.1
Study results.

	Median	P value
Acute studies		
% Change in average daily consumption time	13.2	0.75
% Change in average daily consumption amount	−3.5	1.0
Chronic studies		
% Change in average daily consumption time	86.0	0.02
% Change in average daily consumption amount	−26.4	0.00

accomplished with surgical procedures. There were no device-related complications and the only source of patient morbidity was a wound infection. Additionally, patients did not complain of significant discomfort from electrical stimulation. No patient needed to deactivate their generators with the magnets.

Thus, this initial clinical experience was not as dramatic as that seen in animal experimentation. What is most striking is the absence of side affects from activation of the small sensory fibers of the vagus nerve, the unmyelinated C fibers. In the animal model, it was possible to induce retching and emesis at high currents. Obviously, this would not be desirable for humans, but the absence of any complaints of nausea leads to consideration of whether the energy threshold necessary to activate enough C fibers could be delivered. As a result, a new generation of electrodes that can deliver double the current are awaited before continuing the clinical trial.

Additionally, the work of Dr Mark George

and his colleagues at the Medical University of South Carolina, with functional magnetic resonance imaging, is being followed (see Chapter 4). This group has shown that VNS increases blood flow to areas such as the hypothalamus that are known to control energy regulation. The ability to see subtle changes in these areas will hopefully provide a rational framework to determine optimal stimulation parameters. Unfortunately, it is still not known why VNS is only 60% effective for the treatment of epilepsy. Does it not work in certain patients because they have a different disease, or do they have different anatomy, or is there a technical problem with the signal, electrode or generator? In refractive epilepsy, where there is no other option, this may be acceptable. However, in other areas with alternatives, higher levels of effectiveness are necessary. Real-time imaging will provide the best opportunity to answer these difficult questions.

At present, electrical stimulation cannot

compare to gastric bypass; however, there are numerous reasons to continue to pursue this research. While many predict a magic bullet, this is highly unlikely. It is the present authors' belief that the pharmaceutical treatment of obesity will require a cocktail of agents that function via different pathways. Since obesity is a chronic disease these agents will have to be given for a long time period. The combination of lifelong therapy and multiple agents will make undesirable events common. Additionally, while the focus here has been on morbid obesity, there is an entire group who are overweight and desire help but are not severe enough to justify surgery. Certainly, a device with a good safety profile would be very attractive. Furthermore, it is possible that VNS can be used with new agents to provide a synergistic effect with some of the > 100 drugs that are in development and lower either the dose or number of medications required for clinical efficacy.

The desire to eat and the body's counter regulatory system when caloric intake is reduced, makes the treatment of obesity quite a difficult task. While a cautionary tone must be taken with the present authors' early data, it is important to point out that the mean 14% weight loss achieved is double that of pharmaceuticals approved by the Food and Drug Administration for obesity. Thus, while

this technology is still in the early stages, the present authors remain optimistic. The vagus nerve is the link from the abdominal viscera to the brain, i.e. the wiring is in place; the task now is to learn the language and find the signal to mimic.

References

1. Mason EE. Gastric surgery for morbid obesity. Surg Clin North Am 1992; 72:501–13.

2. Gastrointestinal surgery for severe obesity. NIH Consensus Dev Conf Consensus Statement 1991; Am J Clin Nutr 1992; 55:615S–619S.

3. Gonzalez MF, Deutsch JA. Vagotomy abolishes cues of satiety produced by gastric distention. Science 1981; 212:1283–4.

4. Smith GP, Jerome C, Cushin BJ et al. Abdominal vagotomy blocks the satiety effect of cholecystokinin in the rat. Science 1981; 213:1036–7.

5. Ritter RC, Ritter S, Ewart WR, Wingate DL. Capsaicin attenuates hindbrain neuron responses to circulating cholecystokinin. Am J Physiol 1989; 257:R1162–8.

6. Bray GA. Afferent signals regulating food intake. Proc Nutr Soc 2000; 59:373–84.

7. Houpt TR, Houpt KA, Swan AA. Duodenal osmoconcentration and food intake in pigs after ingestion of hypertonic nutrients. Am J Physiol 1983; 245:R181–9.

Vagus nerve stimulation in the current treatment of epilepsy

Dieter Schmidt

7

Introduction

Initial treatment of epilepsy with antiepileptic drugs (AED) is effective in 49% of patients.[1] If seizures in the remaining patients fail to respond to a second AED, the chances for acceptable seizure control with drug therapy are < 5%.[1] Therefore, non-pharmacological treatments, including resective epilepsy surgery, vagus nerve stimulation (VNS) and the ketogenic diet should be considered for patients whose seizures continue despite at least two trials of AED.[2]

When discussing the role of VNS in the treatment of epilepsy, a group of US experts recently came to the following conclusions: 'The degree of improvement in seizure control from VNS remains comparable to that of new antiepileptic drugs, but is lower than that of mesial temporal lobectomy in suitable surgical resection candidates ... The efficacy of VNS in less severely affected populations remains to be evaluated. Nevertheless, sufficient evidence exists to rank vagus nerve stimulation for epilepsy as effective and safe.'[3]

This chapter reviews the place of VNS in the treatment of epilepsy.

Risk–benefit assessment of vagus nerve stimulation (VNS) versus antiepileptic drugs (AEDs)

Insufficient long-term seizure control and side effects limit the clinical benefit of AED treatment. Unfortunately, the introduction of AEDs over the past decade has not significantly reduced the proportion of patients with chronic, drug-refractory epilepsy.[4] This is due to efficacy profiles that are not substantially better than for the older AEDs as well as safety concerns, such as liver failure and aplastic anemia with the use of felbamate; irreversible, concentric visual field defects due to vigabatrin,[5] and severe hypersensitivity reactions with lamotrigine. Because of these and other factors, only about one in three patients remains on long-term treatment with new AEDs after 3 years.[6,7]

The effectiveness of VNS relative to AEDs in patients who do not respond to initial AED treatment is not known due to the lack of randomized, controlled trials that compare VNS and AED in this population. Any comparison, therefore, is indirect and based on the results of separate trials with similar study populations. The efficacy of VNS for epilepsy has been detailed in Chapter 3, and a brief overview of its efficacy and clinical utility is given here.

VNS results in a reduction in seizure frequency, attenuation of seizure severity, and positive changes in alertness and mood, and offers the potential for aborted seizures with on-demand stimulation. Each of these effects contribute to the clinical utility of VNS. Seizure reduction has been demonstrated in two double-blind, randomized, active-controlled trials (E03 and E05).[8] In both trials, the primary efficacy analysis was the percentage change in total seizure frequency during treatment with VNS versus a prospective baseline, comparing the two treatment groups: (1) high-stimulation group (30 Hz, 30 seconds on and 5 minutes off, 500 microsecond pulse width, and a maximally tolerated current); (2) low-stimulation group (1 Hz, 30 seconds on and 90–180 minutes off, 130 microsecond pulse width, and a just-perceived current). In the E03 study, the high-stimulation group had a mean reduction in seizure frequency of 24.5%, versus 6.1% for the low-stimulation group ($P = 0.01$). In the E05 study, the between-group difference was 13% (28% versus 15%; $P = 0.039$).

Efficacy appears to improve over time with chronic VNS. In a prospective, 12-month continuation study of 195 patients who completed the E05 study, those patients who received high stimulation during the E05 study continued to receive VNS within recommended settings (0.25–3.5 mA, 7–60 seconds on and 1.1–180 minutes off, 20–30 Hz frequency, and 500–750 microsecond pulse width), and patients who were on low stimulation during the double-blind trial were transferred to high stimulation (as defined for the E05 study) during the 12-month evaluation period. The primary efficacy outcome measure was the percentage change in total seizure frequency at 3 and 12 months. At 3 months, the median reduction was 34% relative to the 3-month pre-implantation baseline; at 12 months, it was 45% ($P = 0.0001$, 12 versus 3 months). Twenty per cent of patients sustained 75% reductions in seizure frequency during the first year of treatment. Therefore, the efficacy of VNS appeared to improve during the 12 months following the completion of the E05 study.[9] Limitations of this open-study design are discussed in detail elsewhere in this book. Most importantly, adjustment of AEDs may confound the specific contribution of VNS in these patients and ongoing therapy with VNS was unblinded.

Additional supportive evidence of clinical improvement with continued VNS comes from the voluntary patient registry program sponsored by the device manufacturer. When 1518 patients from the registry were assessed by their physicians 12 months after implantation, the median seizure reduction was 58%, as compared to 49% at 3 months. In addition, 20% of patients had a seizure reduction $\geq 90\%$ at 12 months, which was four times greater than at 3 months.[10]

The long-term outcome of VNS following 29 months of treatment was studied in a separate group of 15 patients with refractory partial epilepsy. The mean stimulation output was 2.25 mA. Four patients (27%) were completely seizure free for ≥ 12 months; in one patient, one AED was tapered; in 10 patients, drug treatment was unchanged; and in four patients, one AED was added. The data from this small series is consistent with the other available data and suggests that VNS remains effective during long-term treatment of patients with medically refractory partial epilepsy.[11]

Another outcome measure for assessing the efficacy of epilepsy therapy is the number needed to treat. Although not free of methodological weaknesses, it provides a graphic overview of how many patients have to be treated until one patient achieves $\geq 50\%$ seizure reduction. Assuming a 10% placebo response, Chadwick[12] calculated the number needed to be treated with VNS to be four to seven patients (95% confidence interval). The corresponding figures for new AED as derived from placebo-controlled add-on trials are shown in Figure 7.1.[13]

The E03 and E05 trials did not include formal evaluations of mood, though several investigators noted mood improvements in their patients.[14,15] More recently, data from 125 patients entered into a patient registry sponsored by the device manufacturer were analyzed for patient-perceived changes in mood, alertness and memory after 12 months of stimulation. Increased alertness was noted

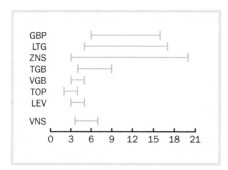

Figure 7.1
Number of patients needed to be treated to achieve a seizure reduction of 50% or more over placebo. Indirect comparisons from placebo-controlled add-on trials and of active-controlled trials of vagus nerve stimulation (VNS).[13]

by 62% of patients, 32% reported improved mood and 24% better memory.[16] Recently published retrospective data from Germany[17] and a prospective study from the US[18] suggest that VNS reduces depressive symptoms in patients with epilepsy. These improvements did not correlate with changes in seizure frequency, suggesting that the antidepressive effect of VNS may be independent of its anticonvulsant effect.

If no improvement in seizure frequency or severity is seen after 2 years of adequate VNS treatment, the generator should be shut off for several months to confirm that no improvement had occurred during stimulation (in which case neither seizure severity or frequency would worsen once stimulation stops). If this is the case, the generator should

then be removed. Typically, the electrodes are left in place in order to avoid injury to the vagus nerve, though successful removal of the electrodes has recently been reported.[19]

Comparing the adverse event profiles of VNS and AEDs is problematic, because patients treated with VNS often receive one or more AEDs, and a number of factors may influence the tolerability and safety of AEDs.[20] With regard to AEDs, 98 of 470 newly treated patients (24%) discontinued their first monotherapy treatment because of intolerable side effects and idiosyncratic reactions.[1] Patients with chronic epilepsy are often exposed to AED polytherapy and may have higher rates of side effects that impair quality of life. Hypersensitivity reactions to AEDs occur in 5–8% of newly treated patients, and teratogenicity is a problem in up to 10% of AED-exposed pregnancies. Up to 1% of patients experience AED-induced disease (Table 7.1).[21]

By comparison, VNS-associated adverse events typically occur only during stimulation, lessen over time, and may be reduced or eliminated with parameter adjustments (as detailed elsewhere in this book). After 1 year of VNS treatment, 29% of patients reported hoarseness or voice change, 8% cough, 12% paresthesia, and 8% dyspnea. After 3 years of VNS, the figures dropped to 2, 2, 0, and 3%, respectively.[22] In contrast to some AEDs, VNS has not been associated with idiosyncratic reactions or deaths.[16] The rate of sudden unexpected death in epilepsy (SUDEP) does not appear to be increased in patients treated with VNS.[23] It should also be noted in comparing VNS and AEDs that compliance or adherence is not a problem with VNS.

Complications of the VNS implantation procedure include (in declining incidence); infection (1.5%), vocal cord paresis (1%), unilateral facial weakness (1%), and (during the early days of VNS and since corrected) lead breakage. (For a detailed discussion of surgical techniques, see Chapter 2.) Further, during the implantation procedure in the operating room, transient asystole lasting 10–20 seconds has been reported in eight patients out of an estimated total of 7000 implantations (approximately 1.1 per 1000). All incidents occurred during the lead test, which consists of approximately 15 seconds of VNS stimulation at 1.0 mA, 500 microseconds and 20 Hz. Four of the eight patients were implanted, and the generator and the electrodes were removed from the remaining four. All patients received standard treatment and recovered without sequelae.[24,25,28] The cause of this rare event has not been fully determined.

Scarring at the incision sites can vary significantly between patients and is technique dependent. Perioperative adverse events reported by at least 10% of patients in the E03 and E05 trials were pain (29%), coughing (14%), voice changes (13%), chest pain (12%), and nausea (10%).[15,26] Although

a number of stimulation-related adverse events were reported during VNS treatment during the E03 and E05 trials, the only adverse events that occurred significantly more often in the high-stimulation group were dyspnea and voice alteration. Adverse events were judged to be mild and transient in almost all patients (Table 7.2). No cognitive, sedative, visual, affective, or neurological deficits were reported. No relevant changes were seen in hematology or routine chemistry testing.[27]

Given that the vagus nerve innervates the heart, the effects of VNS on cardiac rhythm were studied extensively in over 250 patients using Holter monitors. No effects on cardiac rate or rhythm were found compared to baseline.[15] Similarly, no clinically significant cardiac problems have been reported with chronic use,[25,27,28] though VNS at high-stimulation parameters has been shown in five patients to lead to mild bradycardia and decreased heart rate variability.[29]

Chronic VNS does not appear to adversely affect pulmonary function in patients without pulmonary disease.[26] More recently, the effects of VNS on sleep-related breathing in four patients with obstructive sleep apnea (OSA) have been reported.[30] Polysomnography (PSG) before and after 3 months of VNS demonstrated that OSA was exacerbated, and the authors therefore concluded that VNS should be administered with care in patients with pre-existing OSA. As OSA may occur unrecognized in one of three patients with

Table 7.1
Global adverse event profile of therapeutic interventions in epilepsy.[21] In terms of adverse event profile and incidence, vagus nerve stimulation (VNS) has a favorable adverse event profile compared to antiepileptic drugs (AEDs) and resective surgery.

	CBZ	CLB	ESM	FBM	GBP	LEV	LTG	OXC	PB	PHT	TGB	TPM	VPA	VGB	ZON	SURG	VNS
Acute toxicity																	
Sedation	Yes	Yes			Yes	Yes	Yes		Yes	Yes	Yes	Yes		Yes	Yes		
Dizziness	Yes	Yes	Yes		Yes	Yes		Yes	Yes	Yes	Yes	Yes		Yes	Yes		
Seizure aggravation	Yes				Yes		Yes	Yes			Yes			Yes			
Gastrointestinal	Yes		Yes	Yes			Yes	Yes	Yes				Yes		Yes		
Liver failure				Yes									Yes				
Hypersensitivity	Yes		Yes	Yes			Yes	Yes	Yes	Yes							
Chronic toxicity																	
Sedation		Yes	Yes						Yes								
Encephalopathy										Yes	Yes	Yes	Yes				
Visual problems	Yes									Yes				Yes			
Movement disorders	Yes									Yes			Yes				
Behavioral problems				Yes	Yes	Yes			Yes	Yes	Yes	Yes				Yes	
Depression			Yes	Yes	Yes	Yes			Yes	Yes	Yes		Yes	Yes		Yes	
Psychosis			Yes	Yes	Yes	Yes			Yes	Yes				Yes		Yes	
Cerebellar deficits										Yes						Yes	
Neuropathy	Yes									Yes							
Leukopenia	Yes		Yes	Yes						Yes							
Aplastic anemia	Yes		Yes	Yes						Yes							
Thrombocytopenia				Yes									Yes				
Megaloblastic anemia									Yes	Yes							
Pancreatitis					Yes								Yes				
Renal disease												Yes					
Cardiac effects																	yes
Skin	Yes								Yes				Yes				
Osteomalacia	Yes								Yes	Yes							
Hyponatremia	Yes							Yes									
Weight problems													Yes	Yes	Yes		

Table 7.1 (continued)

Worse cognition	Yes	Yes														Yes	
Memory problems																Yes	
Teratogenicity	Yes	Yes	Yes														
Immunological	Yes	Yes	Yes														
AED–AED interactions	Yes		Yes		Yes	Yes	Yes	Yes	Yes								
AED–drug interactions	Yes		Yes		Yes	Yes	Yes	Yes	Yes								
Surgical treatment																	
Asystole																	Yes*
Dyspnea, cough																	Yes
Hoarseness, vocal cord paralysis																	Yes
Neck discomfort, paresthesia																	Yes
Dysphagia																	Yes
Anesthesiological and surgical complications																Yes	Yes
Sum of adverse events	13	5	8	8	5	5	5	7	18	20	5	8	11	9	5	7	6

CBZ, Carbamazepine; CLB, clobazam or clonazepam; ESM, ethosuximide; FBM, felbamate; GBP, gabapentin; LEV, levetiracetam; LTG, lamotrigine; OXC, oxcarbazepine; PB, phenobarbital; PHT, phenytoin; PRM, primidone; SURG, resective epilepsy surgery; TGB, tiagabine; TPM, topiramate; VPA, valproate; VGB, vigabatrin; VNS, vagus nerve stimulation; Yes, the adverse event has been reported in a number of patients in association with the intervention; ZON, zonisamide. *During intraoperative lead test (see text).

Table 7.2
Advantages and disadvantages of vagus nerve stimulation (VNS).

Advantages	Disadvantages
1. No invasive preoperative evaluation or craniotomy is required for VNS 2. Reduces the number of seizures by at least half in approximately 50% in patients with refractory partial epilepsy and Lennox–Gastaut syndrome 3. Patient may have self-control over severe seizures by magnet 4. Treatment compliance is assured 5. No interactions with anticonvulsants 6. Well tolerated and accepted by patients	1. Only a small minority of patients become seizure free 2. Prior to implantation, the effects are difficult to predict 3. Requires battery change after device end-of-service 4. During stimulation voice changes and dyspnea upon exertion may occur

medically refractory partial epilepsy,[31] it would seem prudent to take a history for possible OSA in candidates for VNS and obtain PSG in appropriate patients prior to implantation. In patients with minimal or mild sleep apnea, increasing off time (e.g. 5 minutes instead of 3 minutes) may prevent the exacerbation of OSA.[30] If reduced VNS stimulation compromises seizure control, or if OSA is moderate or severe, treatment of OSA may be advisable before considering VNS therapy. In fact, improving OSA may also be beneficial for seizure control in patients with coexisting OSA and epilepsy. In patients without OSA, VNS may be associated with sleep-related decreases in airflow, and more frequent apneas and hypopneas during stimulation, which are probably not clinically significant.[30]

Short-wave diathermy, microwave diathermy and therapeutic ultrasound diathermy are generally contraindicated for patients with implanted neurostimulation systems, although to date no diathermy related adverse events have been reported in association with VNS treatment. Diathermy could theoretically cause heating of the generator or at the electrode–vagus nerve interface in the neck, potentially resulting in temporary or permanent nerve, tissue, or vascular damage.

As approximately 0.5% of all pregnancies occur in women with epilepsy, and about 20% of female patients with epilepsy are of childbearing age, it is important to assess the safety of VNS during pregnancy. In one report, eight women were treated with adjunctive VNS during pregnancy. The outcomes were normal in five patients, including one pair of twins; one unplanned pregnancy ended in an elective abortion; one pregnancy was terminated because of abnormal in-utero fetal development; and one patient reported a spontaneous abortion, though in this case the actual pregnancy was not confirmed. These latter two outcomes were thought to be related to the natural histories of the patients' disorders or to concomitant AED treatment that the women were receiving simultaneously with VNS.[32]

In summary, VNS is well tolerated. Stimulation-associated adverse events are usually mild and reversible upon reduction of the output current or stimulus duration. In addition, patients accommodate many of the adverse events after several months of treatment. Although head-to-head studies have not been done, VNS appears to be better tolerated and safer than many AEDs, and, in contrast to AEDs, VNS is not associated with chronic systemic complications. Experience in pregnancy is limited.

Risk–benefit assessment of vagus nerve stimulation (VNS) versus other non-pharmacological adjunctive treatment

Non-pharmacological treatments for patients who do not achieve satisfactory seizure control from AEDs, or who have significant adverse

effects,[33] include VNS, brain surgery, and the ketogenic diet.

Surgical resection of epileptogenic tissue is an important treatment option for patients with intractable, medication-resistant partial epilepsy, and up to 70% of seizure patients become seizure free.[34] The efficacy of resective surgery for drug-resistant temporal lobe epilepsy was recently assessed for the first time in a randomized controlled trial comparing immediate temporal lobe surgery with continued medical treatment versus optimized medical treatment alone. At 1 year, 38% of patients who underwent surgery were free of seizures that impaired awareness, compared to 8% in the group receiving medication alone ($P < 0.001$). This trial demonstrated that the combination of surgery with AED treatment is more effective at controlling seizures in selected patients than drug treatment alone.[35]

The efficacy of resective surgery in this trial was lower than the 70% reported in uncontrolled clinical observations.[36] However, four of the 40 patients assigned to the surgical arm of the study did not actually undergo surgery, so 64% of those actually undergoing surgery were free of disabling seizures. Other possible explanations for the discrepancy are: (1) the controlled trial design is a more stringent test than clinical observations; (2) the surgical outcome may continue to improve during longer post-surgical follow-up than was carried out in the trial.

Most experts agree that patients who

become seizure free after surgery, and remain so for several years after complete withdrawal of their medication, are cured of their epilepsy. Only a minority of patients, however, appear to meet this definition of a cure. In one recent retrospective study, efforts to completely discontinue AEDs in patients who were seizure free after surgery resulted in seizure relapse in 30 of 84 patients (36%).[37] When drugs were tapered but not withdrawn, seizures recurred in 13 of 96 patients (14%), and in 30 patients where drug treatment was not changed, two patients (7%) experienced a recurrence of seizures. These findings suggest that most patients undergoing epilepsy surgery require ongoing drug treatment.[38]

The complications and discomforts of epilepsy surgery are well known and include the risk of presurgical testing, including withdrawal of AEDs, if necessary, and invasive electroencephalogram (EEG) monitoring with intracranial electrode placement, if required. Although most patients benefit from surgery, and surgical mortality is extremely rare, complications in a large series of 215 patients included infection of bone flap (1.3%), mild hemiparesis (0.9%), hemianopia (0.4%), transient cranial nerve palsies (3.2%), difficulty with verbal memory (8.8%), postoperative psychosis (2.3%) or depression (5.5%), and postoperative language difficulties (3.7%).[39] In a series from Germany, temporal lobe epilepsy led to a significant decline in memory function in 51% of patients

undergoing left selective amygdalohippocampectomy and in 32% of patients after right-sided surgery.[40]

It has been estimated that only up to 5% of patients with drug-refractory epilepsy who are surgical candidates actually undergo resective epilepsy surgery due to the limited availability of qualified comprehensive epilepsy centers.[36] Consequently, the large majority of patients with drug-refractory epilepsy are in need of other non-pharmacological treatment modalities.[36] VNS offers several advantages over resective epilepsy surgery. VNS requires only relatively minor surgery, without any ablation, and its effect is adjustable and reversible. Beneficial cognitive effects have been reported in association with chronic VNS. The remaining major non-pharmacological therapy is the ketogenic diet, first developed 80 years ago, which is primarily used to decrease seizure frequency in children with severe types of epilepsy.[41]

Place of vagus nerve stimulation (VNS) in the treatment of epilepsy

New-onset or early epilepsy

AEDs are clearly the initial treatment of choice for patients with new-onset or early epilepsy, though the available evidence suggests AEDs are anti-ictal rather than anti-epileptogenic.[38]

There are no data to support the use of

VNS in this patient group. Not surprisingly, therefore, when asked about initial treatment choice for any type of epilepsy, US epilepsy specialists viewed VNS as a treatment one would rarely use or use only in special circumstances.[42]

Chronic, drug-refractory epilepsy

A substantial proportion of patients with newly treated seizures turn out to have medically refractory epilepsy. Indeed, for patients who do not respond to drug treatment within the first 2 years of therapy, the long-term outlook is currently uncertain at best and grim for most.[43] This problem may be more widespread than generally appreciated by neurologists. When 1023 individuals with epilepsy responded to a community based questionnaire, 89% reported that their seizures were, in their estimation, at least somewhat controlled, yet 57% reported having suffered more than one seizure in the preceding year. The authors concluded: 'Despite advances in epilepsy therapy, freedom from seizures and optimal quality of life eludes many.'[44,45] In addition, there is a growing concern that chronic epilepsy is a progressive disorder, at least in some patients (e.g. those with mesial temporal lobe epilepsy), and that recurring seizures may possibly also contribute to a progressive decline in neuropsychological status.[46]

In a recent survey of 51 US epilepsy

experts, an evaluation for epilepsy surgery was recommended for patients with symptomatic partial epilepsy after failure of two monotherapies and a combination of two adequate drugs.[42] In addition, VNS was recommended for treatment of symptomatic partial epilepsy after failure of two monotherapies, or three combination therapies, or before starting any three-drug regimen.

Similarly, Benbadis et al[47] suggested a role for VNS in patients who were determined not to be surgical candidates based on presurgical evaluation and also in those for whom resective surgery had failed (Figure 7.2).

For idiopathic generalized epilepsy, the experts recommended VNS after failure of three monotherapies and three combination therapies; the ketogenic diet achieved a similar position in this ranking. In patients with symptomatic generalized epilepsy, VNS was recommended only after failure of three monotherapies, three combination therapies, the ketogenic diet, and a fourth combination treatment, but before starting resective epilepsy surgery evaluation.[42]

Although the value of VNS for treating patients with refractory generalized epilepsy is less well documented, it may still be an option in refractory Lennox–Gastaut syndrome (LGS), and in related syndromes of catastrophic epilepsies in childhood and adolescence. If standard treatment with three or more adequate AED does not achieve

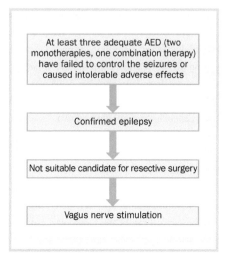

Figure 7.2
Decision algorithm for vagus nerve stimulation (VNS) in the treatment of epilepsy.

sufficient seizure control, or proves to be intolerable, VNS may be tried.[48] Based on controlled trials in partial epilepsy and clinical observations in refractory LGS, a group of European epilepsy experts recently concluded that VNS is a palliative surgical procedure similar in efficacy to the newer AEDs for patients who cannot be treated sufficiently with existing anticonvulsants or resective epilepsy surgery.[49] In a subgroup of patients from study E04 who had generalized seizures exclusively, and only generalized epileptiform activity or generalized slowing in the EEG and unchanged AED treatment, the effectiveness of VNS during the first 3 months was

compared to a 1-month baseline before implantation. The open data from this short-term clinical study suggest that VNS may have a beneficial effect on seizure frequency in children (4 years of age and above), adolescents, and adults with refractory generalized epilepsy.[48]

In a recent evaluation of treatment for LGS, one of the major syndromes of symptomatic generalized epilepsies, VNS was recommended before surgical callosal resection was considered in patients both above and below 5 years of age because VNS offers a better risk–benefit assessment given the significant postoperative complications of callosal resection (Figures 7.3–7.5). In addition, callosal resection remains an option when VNS has not been sufficiently effective.[50]

Conclusions

VNS is a well-tolerated, effective, and safe therapy for medically refractory epilepsy. Efficacy for partial seizures that cannot be treated sufficiently with existing AEDs or resective epilepsy surgery appears to be similar to the newer AEDs. In addition, clinical observations suggest that VNS treatment may also be useful in patients with refractory LGS and related syndromes.

Individualized risk–benefit assessment of initial and subsequent AEDs is the key to treatment. Patients with epilepsy should be

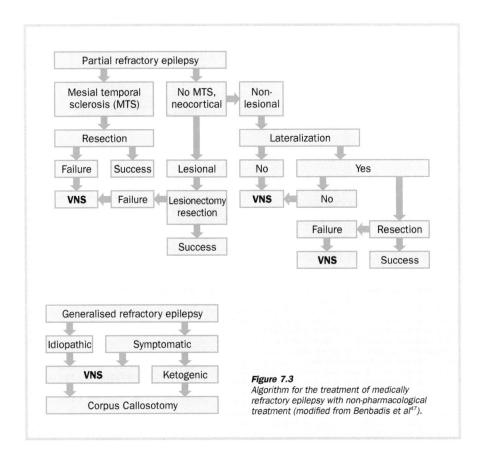

Figure 7.3
Algorithm for the treatment of medically refractory epilepsy with non-pharmacological treatment (modified from Benbadis et al[47]).

counseled about all of their therapeutic options, including VNS, in order to help them make informed choices. When VNS is discussed, it is important to be sure patients understand that:

• VNS will likely not lead to complete seizure control;

• it may take 6–24 months to fully benefit from VNS;

• the generator may be visible or palpable;

• special precautions need to be taken with magnetic resonance imaging (MRI) scanning due to the implanted device;

• visits for individual titration and fine tuning of parameters are required.

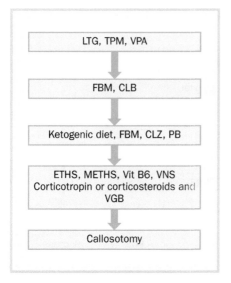

Figure 7.4
Algorithm for the treatment of Lennox–Gastaut syndrome and related syndromes in patients below 5 years of age (modified from Schmidt and Bourgeois[50]). For abbreviations see Table 7.1. ETHS, ethosuximide; METH, methsuximide.

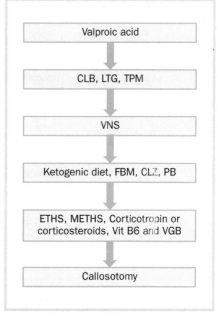

Figure 7.5
Algorithm for the treatment of Lennox–Gastaut syndrome and related syndromes in patients above 5 years of age (modified from Schmidt and Bourgeois[50]). For abbreviations see Tables 7.1 and 7.2.

In the foreseeable future, AED will remain the mainstay of epilepsy treatment. If a satisfactory outcome is not attained early on, i.e. after several appropriate courses of AED, then it is reasonable to consider resective surgery, VNS or the ketogenic diet (in children). In refractory temporal lobe epilepsy, resective surgery is usually the first non-pharmacological option; if the individual risk–benefit of surgery is not favorable, however, VNS is an effective, well-tolerated and less invasive approach.

References

1. Kwan P, Brodie MJ. Early identification of refractory epilepsy. N Engl J Med 2000; 342:314–19.

2. Brodie MJ. Do we need any more new antiepileptic drugs? Epilepsy Res 2001; 45:3–6.

3. Fisher RS, Handforth A. Reassessment: vagus nerve stimulation for epilepsy? A report of the therapeutics and technology assessment

subcommittee of the American Academy of Neurology. Neurology 1999; 53:666–9.

4. Schmidt D. Clinical impact of new antiepileptic drugs. Epilepsy Res 2002; 50(1&2):21–32.

5. Perucca E, Beghi E, Dulac O et al. Assessing risk to benefit ratio in antiepileptic drug therapy. Epilepsy Res 2000; 41:107–39.

6. Krakow K, Walker M, Otoul C, Sander JWAS. Long-term continuation of levetiracetam in patients with refractory epilepsy. Neurology 2001; 56:1772–4.

7. Lhatoo SD, Wong ICK, Polizzi G, Sander JWAS. Long-term retention rates of lamotrigine, gabapentin, and topiramate in chronic epilepsy. Epilepsia 2000; 41:1592–6.

8. Schachter SC. Efficacy, safety and tolerability: clinical trials. In: Schachter SC, Schmidt D (eds). Vagus Nerve Stimulation. (Martin Dunitz: London, 2001) 51–64.

9. DeGiorgio CM, Amar A, Apuzzo MLJ. Surgical anatomy, implantation technique, and operative complications. In: (Schachter SC, Schmidt D, eds) Vagus Nerve Stimulation. (Martin Dunitz: London, 2001) 31–50.

10. Schachter SC. VNS: efficacy, safety, and tolerability. Proceedings of the International VNS Symposium & Workshop CD ROM, September 6–9, 2001 Sintra (Portugal).

11. Vonck K, Boon P, D'Have M et al. Long-term results of vagus nerve stimulation in refractory epilepsy. Seizure 1999; 8:328–34.

12. Chadwick D. Vagal nerve stimulation for epilepsy. Lancet 2001; 357:1726–7.

13. Robinson G. Paediatric experience and some conclusions. Proceedings of the International

VNS Symposium & Workshop CD ROM, September 6–9, 2001 Sintra (Portugal).

14. Ben-Menachem E, Manon-Espaillat R, Ristanovic R et al. Vagus nerve stimulation for treatment of partial seizures: 1. A controlled study of effect on seizures. Epilepsia 1994; 35:616–26.

15. Handforth A, DeGiorgio CM, Schachter SC et al. Vagus nerve stimulation therapy for partial-onset seizures: a randomized active-control trial. Neurology 1998; 51:48–55.

16. Cyberonics, Inc., data on file, 2002.

17. Elger G, Hoppe C, Falkai P et al. Vagus nerve stimulation is associated with mood improvements in epilepsy patients. Epilepsy Res 2000; 42:203–10.

18. Harden CL, Pulver MC, Nikolov B et al. Effect of vagus nerve stimulation on mood in adult epilepsy patients. Neurology 1999; 52(Suppl 2):A238 (abstract).

19. Espinosa J, Aiello MT, Naritoku DK. Revision and removal of stimulation electrodes following long-term therapy with the vagus nerve stimulator. Surg Neurol 1999; 51:659–64.

20. Pirmohamed M, Park BK. Genetic susceptibility to adverse drug reactions. Trends Pharmacol Sci 2001; 22:298–305.

21. Schmidt D, Elger CE. Praktische Epilepsiebehandlung, 2nd edn. (Thieme: Stuttgart, 2002.)

22. Schachter SC. Efficacy, safety, and tolerability. In: (Schachter SC, Schmidt D, eds) Vagus Nerve Stimulation (2nd edition) (Martin Dunitz: London, 2003) 49–66.

23. Annegers JF, Coan SP, Hauser WA et al. Epilepsy, vagal nerve stimulation by the NCP System, mortality, and sudden unexpected, unexplained death. Epilepsia 1998; 39:206–12.

24. Andriola MR, Rosenzweig T, Vlay S. Vagus nerve stimulator (VNS): induction of asystole during implantation with subsequent successful stimulation. Epilepsia 2000; 41(Suppl 7):223.

25. Asconape JJ, Moore DD, Zipes DP et al. Bradycardia and asystole with the use of vagus nerve stimulation for the treatment of epilepsy: a rare complication of intraoperative testing. Epilepsia 1999; 40:1452–4.

26. The Vagus Nerve Stimulation Study Group. A randomized controlled trial of chronic vagus nerve stimulation for treatment of medically refractory seizures. Neurology 1995; 45:224–30.

27. Schachter SC, Saper CB. Vagus nerve stimulation. Epilepsia 1998; 39:677–86.

28. Tatum WO 4th, Moore DB, Stecker MM et al. Ventricular asystole during vagus nerve stimulation for epilepsy in humans. Neurology 1999; 52:1267–9.

29. Frei MG, Osorio I. Left vagus nerve stimulation with the neurocybernetic prosthesis has complex effects on heart rate and on its variability in humans. Epilepsia 2001; 42:1007–16.

30. Malow BA, Edwards J, Marzec M et al. Effects of vagus nerve stimulation on respiration during sleep: a pilot study. Neurology 2000; 55:1450–4.

31. Malow BA, Levy K, Maturen K, Bowes R. Obstructive sleep apnea is common in medically refractory epilepsy patients. Neurology 2000; 55:1002–7.

32. Ben-Menachem E, Ristanovic R, Murphy J. Gestational outcomes in epilepsy patients receiving vagus nerve stimulation. Epilepsia 1998; 39(Suppl 6):S180.

33. Aiken SP, Brown WM. Treatment of epilepsy: existing therapies and future developments. Front Biosci 2000; 5:E124–E152.

34. Foldvary N, Bingaman WE, Wyllie E. Surgical treatment of epilepsy. Neurol Clin 2001; 19:491–515.

35. Wiebe S, Blume WT, Girvin JP, Eliasziw M. A randomized, controlled trial of surgery for temporal-lobe epilepsy. N Engl J Med 2001; 345:311–18.

36. Engel J. Surgical Treatment of the Epilepsies, 2nd edn. (Raven Press: New York, 1993.)

37. Schiller Y, Cascino GD, So EL, Marsh WR. Discontinuation of antiepileptic drugs after successful epilepsy surgery. Neurology 2000; 54:346–9.

38. Schachter SC. Current evidence indicates that antiepileptic drugs are anti-ictal, not antiepileptic. Epilepsy Res 2002; 50(1&2):67–70.

39. Salanova V, Markand O, Worth R. Temporal lobe epilepsy surgery: outcome, complications, and late mortality rate in 215 patients. Epilepsia 2002; 43:170–4.

40. Gleissner U, Helmstaedter C, Schramm J, Elger CE. Memory outcome after selective amygdalohippocampectomy. A study in 140 patients with temporal lobe epilepsy. Epilepsia 2002; 43:87–95.

41. Lefevre F, Aronson N. Ketogenic diet for the treatment of refractory epilepsy in children: a systematic review of efficacy. Pediatrics 2000; 105:E46.

42. Karceski S, Morrell M, Carpenter D. The Expert Consensus Guideline Series; treatment of epilepsy. Epilepsy Behav 2001; 2:A1–A50.

43. Hauser WA. The natural history of drug resistant epilepsy: epidemiological

considerations. Epilepsy Res Suppl 1992; 5:25–8.

44. Fisher R, Vickrey BG, Gibson P et al. The impact of epilepsy from the patient's perspective. I. Descriptions and subjective perceptions. Epilepsy Res 2000; 41:39–51.

45. Fisher R, Vickrey BG, Gibson P et al. The impact of epilepsy from the patient's perspective. II. Views about therapy and health care. Epilepsy Res 2000; 41:53–61.

46. Sutula TP, Hermann B. Progression in mesial temporal lobe epilepsy. Ann Neurol 1999; 45:553–6.

47. Benbadis SR, Tatum WO, Vale FL. When drugs don't work: an algorithmic approach to medically intractable epilepsy. Neurology 2000 Dec 26;55(12):1780–4.

48. Labar D, Murphy J, Tecoma E and the E04 VNS Study Group. Vagus nerve stimulation for medication-resistant generalized epilepsy. Neurology 1999; 52:1510–12.

49. Schmidt D, Elger CE, Stefan H et al. Role of vagus nerve stimulation in the treatment of epilepsy. Nervenheilkunde 1999; 18:558–61 (in German).

50. Schmidt D, Bourgeois, B. A risk–benefit assessment of therapies for Lennox–Gastaut syndrome. Drug Saf 2000; 22:467–77.

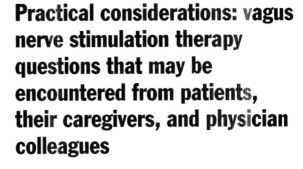

Practical considerations: vagus nerve stimulation therapy questions that may be encountered from patients, their caregivers, and physician colleagues

Christi N Heck and Dieter Schmidt

Introduction

The goal of this chapter is to provide readers with a spectrum of questions patients and physicians may have about the current use of vagus nerve stimulation (VNS) therapy in epilepsy. An attempt has been made to avoid repeating material from earlier chapters, but some overlap is unavoidable.

Patients

What is VNS therapy?

In humans, VNS therapy usually refers to the stimulation of the left vagus nerve with a commercial device, the VNS therapy system, which was developed and is marketed by Cyberonics, Inc. (Houston, Texas). As delivered via this mechanism, VNS therapy is similar to the very common practice of implanting cardiac pacemakers. In both devices, a subcutaneously implanted generator sends an electrical signal through a subcutaneous lead to electrodes attached to the target organ. In contrast to cardiac pacemakers, in which the heart is directly stimulated, VNS therapy delivers signals to the brain through two bipolar electrodes wrapped around the cervical portion of the vagus nerve, one of the cranial extensions of the brain. A programmable bipolar pulse generator implanted in the left chest wall produces the signals and sends them through a subcutaneous lead to the two vagus nerve electrodes. The Model 101 generator is the size of a pocket watch – 53 mm in diameter, 48 mm in height, 10.4 mm in thickness and 36 g in weight. The newer Model 102 generator is 52.2 mm in diameter, 6.9 mm in thickness and 25 g in weight. To minimize the risk of tissue and nerve damage, the generator uses high-frequency stimulation.

Implantation of the generator in the chest wall (similar to a cardiac pacemaker) and subcutaneous placement of the cervical leads are accomplished in one surgical session usually lasting no more than 1 hour. Although local anesthesia may be feasible in principle, most patients receive general anesthesia to control for possible seizure activity that might occur during the procedure. The implantation is usually performed by neurosurgeons, vascular surgeons, or ear, nose and throat specialists familiar with the anatomy of the vagus nerve adjacent to the carotid artery in the neck.

After implantation and intraoperative lead testing, the physician or nurse specialist programs the device during outpatient visits. Placing the VNS therapy programming wand over the generator implanted in the chest allows non-invasive telemetric communication between the software, laptop computer, and generator.

Furthermore, each patient is given a magnet that, when held over the generator, temporarily shuts off the generator, thereby stopping the VNS therapy for as long as the magnet is held over the site. When the magnet is removed, normal operation resumes. Also, early during an aura or seizure, the patient or caregiver may swipe the magnet over the generator in the chest to activate additional stimulation and potentially abort an impending seizure.

Why is the device implanted on the left side?

VNS therapy is traditionally performed on the left vagus nerve. Several suggestions have been made to explain the preference for the left over the right vagus nerve for stimulation. First, the left and right nerves may carry different information. The right vagus nerve is thought to be more closely involved in the regulation of the cardiac atria and the left with cardiac ventricular function. Also, the left vagus nerve is stimulated below the cardiac branches of the vagus nerve. This may explain why cardiac function is unaffected by routine VNS therapy to the left vagus nerve. A second theory holds that cardiac response is more a function of VNS therapy parameters than the choice of the left or right nerve: animal experimentation has not clarified this issue.[1]

Whatever the reason, stimulation is traditionally performed on the left vagus nerve without any adverse events during VNS therapy[2] – patients who experience transient asystole during initial intraoperative stimulation for lead testing will be discussed separately.

How are seizures reduced?

Broad attempts to explain the mechanism(s) of pharmacological action aimed at reducing epileptic seizures, especially partial seizures, are conveniently classified into five categories: (1) blocking ion currents (sodium, potassium, calcium) across the membranes of nerve cells; (2) increasing brain inhibition by enhancing the gamma-aminobutyric acid (GABA)-ergic neurotransmission; (3) attenuation of glutamatergic excitatory neurotransmission; (4) modifying the monoaminergic regulation of seizure control; and (5) unknown.

The question of how VNS therapy may modulate seizure control has not been clarified. Traditionally, the vagus nerve has been considered to be a parasympathetic efferent nerve regulating autonomic functions such as heart rate and gastric tone. However, the vagus nerve, also called the Xth cranial nerve, is actually a mixed nerve composed of about 80% afferent sensory fibers carrying information to the brain from the head, neck and abdomen. The sensory afferent cell bodies reside in the nodose ganglion and relay information to the nucleus tractus solitarius (NTS) and onward to many brain areas, including the frontal lobe and limbic system. Walker et al[3] investigated how the NTS might be involved in the regulation of seizure control. They found that microinjecting the NTS with either GABA or a glutamate antagonist blocked experimental seizures in rats. The NTS has direct connections to the locus coeruleus (LC) and the forebrain in rats. Krahl et al[4] showed that destroying the LC eliminated the ability of VNS therapy to suppress seizures in rats. The LC is the site of many norepinephrine-containing neurons that have important connections to the limbic system, including the amygdala, the hypothalamus and the orbitofrontal cortex. These areas have been linked to the modulation of seizure control, mood and anxiety.

These findings suggest a return to the monoamine theory of epilepsy, which was popular before the current GABA and glutamate theories. Alternative theories do exist; nevertheless, these findings allow speculation concerning how VNS reduces seizures via modulation of monoaminergic, GABA-ergic and glutaminergic neurons. Future studies will have to test these mechanistic hypotheses. Chapter 1 of this volume provides a more detailed explanation of the VNS therapy mechanism of action.

How is the clinical utility of VNS therapy assessed?

In patients with epilepsy, VNS therapy has been shown to lead to seizure reduction, a reduction in seizure severity, the ability to abort seizures using a magnet, and a positive effect on alertness and mood. All of these factors contribute to the clinical utility of VNS. Seizure reduction has been shown in a total of five controlled trials, notably E03 and E05; the other effects have emerged from clinical observational studies.

All the effects of VNS therapy take time to work. However, if no improvement is seen in any of these areas after 2 years of adequate use of VNS, then the stimulation should be set at 0 mA for several months to confirm lack of efficacy. If lack of efficacy is confirmed, the generator can be safely removed with local anesthesia administered to the patient (similar to removal of a cardiac pacemaker). The electrodes are often left in place. Although the successful removal of electrodes has been reported, such a procedure requires general anesthesia, and a lengthy and tedious effort on the part of the surgeon.

Is the effect maintained?

The short answer is yes. The long-term effect of VNS therapy has been documented in multiple clinical trials, as well as from the VNS therapy patient outcome registry. When 1864 patients from the registry were assessed by their physicians 12 months after implantation, the median seizure reduction was 56% (June 30, 2002 data from the voluntary registry organized by Cyberonics, Inc.). This is an improvement over the results, from the same registry, of a median seizure reduction of 45% at 3 months. After 12 months of treatment, 19% of these patients had a 90% or greater seizure reduction compared with baseline. This change reflects an increase in response between 3 and 12 months of treatment.

What are the chances for long-term results in cases of medically refractory epilepsy?

The best evidence for long-term outcomes in cases of medically refractory patients is that obtained by the XE5 Open-label Treatment of Refractory Partial-onset Seizures Using Vagus Nerve Stimulation: Safety and Efficacy follow-up study to the E05 clinical trial.[3] In this study, the 195 patients who completed the E05 protocol were offered open-label follow-up. Of the 195 patients who enrolled, 168 completed this follow-up trial. Patients were followed for an additional 18 months beyond the 3-month E05 study for efficacy and safety. Of the 27 patients who were discontinued from this long-term follow-up, 21 demonstrated lack of efficacy, three had adverse events, one was lost to follow-up and two died. Patients in the high-stimulation group of the E05 study acute phase experienced a mean seizure frequency reduction of 27.9% as compared with baseline. Patients in the XE5 study who continued from the high-stimulation group achieved 37.1% mean seizure reduction at 6 months of treatment. The low-stimulation group from the E05 study took longer to reach the effectiveness rates of their high-stimulation group counterparts. However, the mean per cent seizure reduction continued to improve with time to 57.5% seizure reduction at 27 months (21 patients).

Can VNS therapy slow the progression of epilepsy?

The progression of disease in chronic partial epilepsy is a serious clinical problem that often leads to increased burden of disease, memory disturbances and worsening of seizure control. Experiments in amygdala-kindled cats show that VNS may, at least partly, delay components of the kindling process. Amygdala kindling in cats is one of several models to study the effect of interventions on the progression of partial epilepsy.[6] Although it would be premature to extrapolate these animal findings to humans, the results are encouraging and focus attention on the evaluation of the effects of VNS therapy on progression of disease.

What role does VNS therapy play in the treatment of epilepsy?

A 1999 report of the Therapeutics and Technology Assessment Subcommittee of the American Academy of Neurology concluded, 'The degree of improvement in seizure control from VNS remains comparable to that of new antiepileptic drugs (AED)[7] but is lower than that of mesial temporal lobectomy in suitable surgical resection candidates . . .[8] Efficacy of VNS in less severely affected populations remains to be evaluated. Nevertheless, sufficient evidence exists to rank VNS for epilepsy as effective and safe, based on a preponderance of Class I evidence.'[9]

As the understanding of pharmacoresistant epilepsy has recently evolved, the role of VNS therapy has likewise broadened. A recent recommendation states, 'A patient with partial-onset seizures should be considered for VNS therapy if his or her seizures have not responded to two to four trials of appropriate AEDs and he or she is either not a good candidate for surgical resection, or is a good candidate but refuses to undergo intracranial surgery.'[10]

Which treatments should be considered before trying VNS therapy?

Many physicians recommend and use VNS therapy after the failure of two to four adequate trials of AEDs in patients with a verified diagnosis of partial epilepsy, and when resective temporal lobectomy for mesial temporal lobe epilepsy has been excluded as an option.

For what types of epilepsy is VNS safe and effective?

Although VNS therapy is accepted as effective and safe for refractory partial epilepsy, its value for treating patients with refractory generalized epilepsy is less well documented. After 3 months of VNS therapy during the E04 study, a subgroup of 24 patients with exclusively generalized seizures experienced a median seizure reduction of 46%, as compared with baseline, and 11 of patients had a 50% or greater reduction in seizure frequency. The data from this short-term clinical study suggest that VNS therapy may have a beneficial effect on seizure frequency in children, adolescents and adults with refractory, generalized epilepsy.[11]

Will VNS therapy affect alertness, memory, or mood?

The controlled clinical trials E03 and E05 did not include formal evaluations of mood, alertness or memory. During these trials, however, several investigators noted perceived mood improvements in their patients.[2,12] Physicians participating in the Cyberonics-sponsored patient registry submit assessments of their patients' quality of life. After 12

months of VNS therapy, improvements were noted in mood (44%), alertness (61%), and memory (33%). A prospective study by Harden et al,[13] suggests that VNS therapy reduces depressive symptoms in patients with epilepsy; these improvements were also noted in patients who did not benefit from improved seizure control. These data suggest that VNS therapy may have an antidepressant effect on patients independent of the effect on seizures.

Will VNS therapy affect my depression?

The effect of VNS therapy on mood has been of interest since the early human clinical trials. A number of studies have attempted to quantify the effect of VNS therapy on mood in patients with epilepsy. The rationale behind this effort is fourfold: (1) observations in clinical trials of positive mood effects; (2) positron emission tomography evidence of the effect of VNS therapy on blood flow in the limbic region; (3) evidence that anticonvulsants are effective in the treatment of mood disorders; (4) VNS therapy is known to alter monoamine concentrations in cerebral fluid.[1]

Harden et al[13] have demonstrated with a variety of formal scales, including the Hamilton Depression, Cornell Dysthymia Rating Scale and the Beck Depression Inventory, that VNS therapy is associated with mood improvement, independent of whether or not patients were experiencing improved seizure control. Formal evaluations of the efficacy of VNS therapy in the treatment of depression in patients without epilepsy are currently underway. Chapter 5 of this volume describes the clinical results of VNS therapy in depression in greater detail.

How safe is VNS therapy?

A number of stimulation-related adverse events were reported during the clinical trials (E03 and E05). However, the only adverse events that occurred significantly more often in the treatment group were dyspnea and voice alteration. Adverse events were judged to be mild and transient in almost all patients. No cognitive, sedative, visual, affective or neurological deficits were reported. Also, no relevant changes were seen during extensive Holter monitoring, during testing of pulmonary functions, or in hematological or routine chemistry testing.[14] VNS therapy was safe and no deaths occurred during the controlled E03 and E05 trials in a total of 313 patients.

VNS is generally well tolerated, and stimulation-associated adverse events are usually mild, transient and reversible upon reduction of output current and/or signal frequency. Patients typically accommodate many of the adverse events after several months of treatment.

What are the side effects of VNS therapy?

As discussed above, the only significant adverse events noted from the randomized, controlled clinical trials (E03 and E05)[2,15] were voice alteration and shortness of breath. These adverse events were rated as mild or moderate 99% of the time, and occurred only during the treatment, or 'on' phase, of VNS therapy. Other possible side effects may include cough, throat pain and paresthesias over the neck incision site or beneath the chin. Rare events of pain to the external ear canal, jaw, or shoulder have also been reported. These events are signs that the device settings should be modified or reduced. A reduction in output current, signal frequency, or pulse width can help eliminate these discomforts.

Can one become pregnant while implanted with the VNS Therapy System?

Data on gestational outcome of eight women who were receiving adjunctive VNS therapy during pregnancy showed normal outcome in five patients with unremarkable and healthy deliveries, including a pair of twins. One unplanned pregnancy was terminated in an elective abortion and one pregnancy was aborted owing to abnormal in utero fetal development. Although the actual pregnancy was not confirmed, one patient reported a spontaneous abortion. The preliminary conclusions based on available evidence were that VNS therapy does not seem to impair contraceptive measures and is considered safe. The abnormal development and abortion were thought to be related to the natural history or to the underlying AED treatment that the women were receiving in addition to VNS therapy.[16]

Will cell phones (airport systems, microwave ovens, etc.) affect the VNS Therapy System?

A study on the possible impairment of VNS therapy function by the use of cellular phones was performed at the Georgia Tech Research Institute. The result was that the VNS Therapy System exceeds the Food and Drug Administration and the European standards for immunity at communication frequencies by more than a factor of 10. The VNS Therapy System was not affected by any cellular phone, analog or digital. Likewise, proximity and use of microwave ovens is considered safe.

Airport security systems may detect the generator. To avoid embarrassment, it is recommended that patients with the implant carry an identification card providing evidence of the implant and physician information. This identification card also carries an 800 number for Cyberonics, Inc., in the event that further questions need to be addressed.

Is magnetic resonance imaging (MRI) of the brain safe?

As discussed previously, the VNS Therapy System is an implantable device in which two electrodes are wrapped around the vagus nerve to deliver VNS therapy. Patients with refractory partial epilepsy must often undergo MRI scans of the brain. Studies show that the VNS Therapy System is safe and the quality of the diagnostic information is not affected when a send-and-receive head coil is used for MRI.[17,18]

Are treatments such as diathermy safe?

Patients implanted with the VNS Therapy System should not receive shortwave diathermy, microwave diathermy or therapeutic ultrasound diathermy. Diagnostic ultrasound is not included in this contraindication. Implanted products, such as the VNS Therapy System, may reflect or concentrate the energy delivered by diathermy, and the energy may cause heating. Such heating may cause temporary or permanent nerve, tissue or vascular damage.[19]

If VNS therapy does not work, can the generator be removed?

VNS therapy pulse generators have been removed for a variety of reasons, including lack of efficacy and battery replacement. The generator can be removed with ease while the patient is under either general or local anesthesia. This procedure is typically performed without excision of the electrodes. To explant the device for lack of efficacy, the simplest procedure is to remove the generator and leave the electrodes in place. The electrodes have been removed, however, to either replace or revise the leads, as well as to completely remove the device because of lack of efficacy. This procedure has been performed safely even after the electrodes have been implanted for several years. This procedure requires considerable time. It requires tedious work, on the part of the surgeon, as well as great care and familiarity with the safety of the nerve.

What will the scars look like?

Implanting the VNS Therapy System results in two scars. One is on the left neck, either in a horizontal neck fold (preferred) or as a vertical incision, approximately 1.5–2 inches in length. The second is either below the left collar bone or, more commonly, in the fold of the axilla (see Chapter 2 for details).

Will AEDs still be required?

VNS therapy is approved for the treatment of medically intractable partial epilepsy as adjunctive (add-on) therapy. VNS therapy has been associated with reductions in the numbers and dosages of AEDs.[5,20] Commonly, if VNS therapy proves efficacious, individual patients may, under their physicians' guidance, reduce the AED dose, or the number of medications. It is likely that an AED will continue to be needed in conjunction with VNS therapy.

How soon will it be known if VNS therapy works?

Patient response is most commonly seen within the first 3 months of treatment, provided that the patient is receiving stimulation adjustments at least monthly. The initial response is a reduction in the most severe types of seizures such as generalized tonic–clonic seizures. Over the course of approximately 12–18 months, further improvement may be evident. The reason for this improvement is not known but it is likely to be multifactorial: (1) a cumulative effect of treatment over time; and (2) the result of on-going adjustments in output current, signal frequency and signal on and off times.[21]

Must the magnet be used?

Not all patients are able to use the magnet effectively to activate the on-demand mode of VNS therapy; however, using the magnet is not a necessity. VNS therapy is programmed to deliver therapy automatically, around the clock, regardless of whether a patient is capable of using the on-demand mode or not.

Patients who recognize auras and apply the on-demand mode early during the onset of a seizure or aura may be able to abort the oncoming seizure. Such use of the magnet is an added benefit to providing seizure control to the patient. Nonetheless, magnet activation is not the only mechanism by which VNS therapy helps to control seizures. In some patients, the seizure-controlling effects of VNS therapy continue to improve for at least 18 months after implantation.[5]

Physicians

Which patients are appropriate candidates for VNS?

The US FDA has approved the VNS therapy system for use as an adjunctive therapy in reducing the frequency of seizures in adults and adolescents over 12 years of age with partial onset seizures that are refractory to antiepileptic medications. Our clinical experience has shown that VNS therapy can be effective in patients aged younger than 12 years and for other types of seizures. Two large clinical trials (E03 and E05) have been completed to compare the effects of high- and low-dose VNS therapy in patients with complex partial epilepsy. In addition, one open-label follow-up of 124 patients with various epilepsy syndromes (E04) has also been reported. Data from these three studies show that 40–45% of patients with

complex partial seizures, with or without secondary generalization, will experience > 50% seizure reduction over time.[2,11,15–17]

Documentation of its use in other seizure types confirms the broad effect of VNS therapy. For example, in the open-label study (E04), some patients with primary generalized seizures were included (29%) and some also reported >50% seizure reduction.

However, few children participated in the above-mentioned studies. Among children with Lennox–Gastaut syndrome (LGS) or other catastrophic epilepsy types, results of VNS therapy are equivocal, with some centers reporting excellent results, particularly concerning the reduction of generalized tonic–clonic seizures; other centers describe only a few patients benefiting from the treatment.[22,23]

Appropriate candidates for VNS therapy are:

- Patients with partial seizures, especially with simple partial seizures and generalized tonic–clonic seizures as a part of the seizure expression, who are not candidates for epilepsy surgery. Patients should have tried at least two or three AED before being considered for VNS therapy. Some evidence suggests that patients with right-sided lesions might have more favorable responses, but results are not conclusive.
- Patients with primary generalized seizures, especially with uncontrolled generalized

tonic–clonic seizures, despite trials with two or three AED.

- Patients with LGS, especially those with generalized tonic–clonic seizures, and who are not severely mentally retarded (i.e. with an IQ > 30.
- Children (whatever age) with any type of refractory epilepsy. Implantation should be considered before callosotomy.
- All the above-listed patients can be considered for VNS therapy even before completing trials of three AED if they experience unacceptable side effects from medication.

Are there contraindications to VNS therapy?

The VNS therapy system is contraindicated for patients who have undergone bilateral or left cervical vagotomy. Shortwave diathermy, microwave diathermy and therapeutic ultrasound diathermy are contraindicated in patients with the VNS therapy system. Diagnostic ultrasound is not included in this contraindication.

Patients with severe asthma or heart disease, particularly cardiac arrhythmias, should be carefully evaluated when VNS Therapy is under consideration. The primary medical conditions for which VNS therapy would be contraindicated include patients with severe asthma or heart disease, particularly cardiac arrhythmias. Before being

implanted, patients who rely on the quality of their voice for their livelihood should participate in a serious dialogue regarding the side effects on voice. Children with swallowing difficulties may also experience worsening of the swallow during the stimulation 'on' phase. To manage both voice change and swallowing difficulties, patients may choose to use the magnet-controlled 'off' mode while speaking, singing or eating.

Are any pre-operative considerations or studies necessary?

As with any other treatment, a confirmed diagnosis of epilepsy is recommended before pursuing VNS therapy. In addition, each patient should have a preoperative electrocardiogram.

Is there any special postoperative care to consider?

Many patients may be discharged home after same-day surgery. It is important to address with patients and their families the possible effects that general anesthesia may have on seizures, particularly in the intractable epilepsy patient. Thus, if a patient lives alone or has complicated seizures, one overnight hospital stay may be necessary for observation, and intravenous administration of anticonvulsants should a seizure or a cluster of seizures occur post-anesthesia.

What are the operative and perioperative adverse events of surgical implantation of the VNS Therapy System?

Operative and perioperative adverse events during surgical implantation of the VNS Therapy System are unusual. A few instances of infection, vocal cord paresis, Horner's syndrome, unilateral facial weakness, lead breakage, bradycardia and asystole have been reported. The rare occurrence of these events is discussed in Chapter 2.

When does one activate the VNS therapy pulse generator?

The VNS Therapy Physician's Manual states that both the magnet and the programmed stimulation must be 0.0 mA for the first 14 days after implantation. However, some physicians initiate stimulation earlier. Most centers wait to activate the VNS therapy pulse generator until the patient is fully awake, alert, and able to cooperate with swallowing assessments and testing of hoarseness of the voice. Some patients require a week or so postoperatively to allow for discomfort from intubation to resolve. The present authors prefer to see the patients in follow-up 1 week postoperatively and to attempt the initial activation then. Infrequently, patients may still not tolerate activation for an additional week.

How should settings be set initially?

VNS settings must always be comfortable for the patient. The initial recommended settings are 0.25 mA output current, 30 Hz signal frequency, and 500 microseconds pulse width. If the patient tolerates this setting, then the output current may be adjusted upward in 0.25 mA increments to a level that can be sensed by the patient, but is tolerable and does not cause pain in the throat, ear, jaw or shoulder. The recommended initial 'on' and 'off' times are 30 seconds 'on' and 5 minutes 'off.' If a patient has frequent seizures, one may opt to slightly shorten the 'off' time in an effort to 'catch' the seizures early in their onset.

If a patient does not tolerate the initial setting of 0.25 mA at 30 Hz, reducing the signal frequency may improve tolerability. Alternatively, one may choose to reduce the pulse width for comfort to 250 microseconds. If this setting is better tolerated, a challenge with an increase in output current in 0.25 mA increments should be attempted. It should be kept in mind that patients will need time to habituate to VNS therapy. Habituation usually takes 24–48 hours, at which time patients may comment that the stimulus is no longer felt. Such a comment is an indication that the settings may be adjusted upward once again.

If a patient does not respond to VNS therapy after several months, what adjustments can be made to the standard settings in an attempt to achieve a response?

Studies have shown that the response of non-responders may improve by adjusting the duty cycle, i.e. the 'on' and 'off' times. If a patient has been challenged by the traditional settings at maximum-tolerated output currents, but has not achieved significant positive results, a trial of reduction in 'off' time is warranted. This technique, referred to as rapid cycling, has been shown to be useful for a subset of patients in a variety of studies.[21]

How often do patients require outpatient evaluation?

The frequency of visits to the outpatient clinic is dependent upon the severity of the epilepsy and the response to VNS therapy. Patients who demonstrate a positive response may not need to be seen as frequently as those whose treatment may need adjustment every 3–4 weeks to optimize therapy.

How is efficacy evaluated?

Before patients are implanted, it is recommended that they keep a seizure diary and maintain it as VNS therapy is initiated and continued. A 3-month pre-implant diary is usually sufficient to provide enough experience for comparison. The seizure type and duration should also be noted, as the initial effects of VNS therapy are not always reductions in seizure frequency, but attenuation of seizure intensity and duration. These effects can then be compared to the pre-implant seizure diaries to establish efficacy.

Can AED be tapered off?

VNS therapy is indicated as adjunctive therapy for intractable partial epilepsy. As a patient responds to this therapy, polypharmacy may then be simplified. Patients often will tolerate a reduction in the number of AEDs without exacerbation of their seizures, but VNS monotherapy is not recommended.

Future inquiries

How may VNS therapy response be predicted for any given patient?

Prediction of VNS therapy response has been attempted based upon the localization of the seizure focus, right versus left hemisphere, and temporal versus other lobes. However, no clear localization-related predictive scheme has held. The vagus nerve afferents have a wide distribution both cortically and subcortically, making this association difficult. Thus far, it has not been possible to predict responders from non-responders before implantation.

What is the mechanism of antiepileptogenic effects of VNS therapy in humans?

Although the antiepileptic effects of VNS therapy are not completely understood, Chapter 1 of this volume offers an explanation of the mechanism of action.

What are the most efficacious VNS therapy parameters? Do some parameters provide more influence on efficacy than others?

Controlled clinical trials have not addressed optimal parameters of VNS therapy in establishing maximal efficacy. The overall message from much of the recent experience with VNS therapy is that once output current, signal frequency and pulse width have been optimized, changing the duty cycle may improve the efficacy of VNS therapy. Once the above parameters have been adjusted systematically, patients who appear to be poor responders to VNS therapy may demonstrate improved response with more frequent cycling of VNS therapy (a reduction in 'off' time).[21]

Would VNS therapy be an option to consider in place of AEDs in patients with non-refractory epilepsy?

Recent theory claims that early intervention in the treatment of epilepsy may prevent patients

from becoming medically refractory.[24] If this early intervention can be accomplished by VNS therapy as opposed to a variety of AEDs, which may have a multitude of intolerable side effects, patients may have positive outcomes early, with less cost both financially and in terms of cognitive impairment.

Acknowledgement

The authors gratefully acknowledge the contributions of Elinor Ben-Menachem, MD, who authored a chapter similar to this one in the first edition of this book.

References

1. George MS, Sackeim HA, Rush AJ et al. Vagus nerve stimulation: a new tool for brain research and therapy. Biol Psychiatry 2000; 47:287–95.

2. Handforth A, DeGiorgio CM, Schachter SC et al. Vagus nerve stimulation therapy for partial onset seizures: a randomized active control trial. Neurology 1998; 51:48–55.

3. Walker BR, Easton A, Gale K. Regulation of limbic motor seizures by GABA and glutamate transmission in nucleus tractus solitarius. Epilepsia 1999; 40:1051–7.

4. Krahl SE, Clark KB, Smith DC, Browning RA. Locus coeruleus lesions suppress the seizure-attenuating effects of vagus nerve stimulation. Epilepsia 1998; 39:709–14.

5. DeGiorgio CM, Schachter S, Handforth A et al. Prospective long-term study of vagus nerve stimulation for the treatment of refractory seizures. Epilepsia 2000; 41:1195–200.

6. Fernández-Guardiola A, Martínez A, Valdés-Cruz A et al. Vagus nerve prolonged stimulation in cats: effects on epileptogenesis (amygdala electrical kindling); behavioral and electrographic changes. Epilepsia 1999; 40:822–9.

7. Levy RH, Mattson RH, Meldrum BS (eds). Antiepileptic Drugs, 4th edn. (Raven Press: New York, 1995) 1–1120.

8. Engel J Jr. Surgery for seizures. N Engl J Med 1966; 334:647–52.

9. Fisher RS, Handforth A. Reassessment: vagus nerve stimulation for epilepsy? A report of the therapeutics and technology assessment subcommittee of the American Academy of Neurology. Neurology 1999; 53:666–9.

10. Schachter SC. Vagus nerve stimuation therapy summary: five years after FDA approval. Neurology 2002; 59(4):515–20.

11. Labar D, Murphy J, Tecoma E, E04 VNS Study Group. Vagus nerve stimulation for medication-resistant generalized epilepsy. Neurology 1999; 52:1510–12.

12. Ben-Menachem E, Manon-Espaillat R, Ristanovic R et al. Vagus nerve stimulation for treatment of partial seizures. 1. A controlled study on seizures. Epilepsia 1994; 35:616–26.

13. Harden CL, Pulver MC, Ravdin LD et al. A pilot study of mood in epilepsy patients treated with vagus nerve stimulation. Epilepsy Behav 2000; 1:93–9.

14. Schachter SC, Saper CB. Vagus nerve stimulation. Epilepsia 1998; 39:677–86.

15. The Vagus Nerve Stimulation Study Group. A randomized controlled trial of chronic vagus nerve stimulation for treatment of medically intractable seizures. Neurology 1995; 45:224–30.

16. Ben-Menachem E, Ristanovic R, Murphy J. Gestational outcomes in patients with epilepsy receiving vagus nerve stimulation. Epilepsia 1998; 39(Suppl 6):180.

17. Nyenhuis JA, Bourland JD, Foster KS et al. Testing of MRI compatibility of the Cyberonics Model 100 NCP Generator and Model 300 Series lead. Epilepsia 1997; 38(Suppl 8):S140.

18. Benbadis SR, Nyhenhuis J, Tatum WO 4th et al. MRI of the brain is safe in patients implanted with the vagus nerve stimulator. Seizure 2001; 10:512–15.

19. Cyberonics, Inc. Physician's Manual. Vagus Nerve Stimulation System 102. (Cyberonics, Inc., Houston, 2002.)

20. Tatum WO, Johnson KD, Goff S et al. Vagus nerve stimulation and drug reduction. Neurology 2001; 56:561–3.

21. Heck C, Helmers SL, DeGiorgio CM. Vagus nerve stimulation therapy, epilepsy, and device parameters: scientific basis and recommendations for use. Neurology 2002 Sep 24;59(6 Suppl 4):S31–7.

22. Ben-Menachem E, Hellstrom K, Waldton C et al. Evaluation of refractory epilepsy treated with vagus stimulation for up to 5 years. Neurology 1999; 52:1265–7.

23. Lundgren J, Amark P, Blennow G et al. Vagus nerve stimulation in 16 children with refractory epilepsy. Epilepsia 1998; 39:809–13.

24. Renfroe JB, Wheless JW. Earlier use of adjunctive vagus nerve stimulation (VNS) therapy for refractory epilepsy. Neurology 2002; 59:526–30.

Glossary

5-Hydroxyindoleacetic acid
Serotonin metabolite; also called 5-HIAA.

6-Hydroxydopamine
Compound used experimentally to cause norepinephrine depletion.

Active-controlled
A study design in which the control group receives either a standard treatment (comparative active-controlled design) or a treatment that has a lower potential for efficacy (attenuated active-controlled design).

A-fibers
Large-caliber, fast-conducting myelinated nerve fibers.

Amplitude, *see* Pulse amplitude

Anterior nucleus (thalamus)
Nuclear mass located in the anterior part of the thalamus.

Antiepileptic drugs
Compounds used for the pharmacological treatment of epileptic seizures and epilepsy, also called anticonvulsants.

Area postrema
An area located on the dorsal surface of the medulla with extensive nets of capillaries and with walls that lack the tight junctions characteristic of the blood-brain barrier. It receives afferent synapses from the vagus nerve, and projects to the nucleus tractus solitarius and the parabrachial nucleus.

Aspiration
The abnormal movement of food, water, vomit or stomach acid into the lungs. Main risk factor is dysphagia. May result in pneumonia.

Asystole
Absence of heartbeat.

Atrioventricular node
Component of the heart's electrical conduction system that carries the impulse from the atria to the ventricles.

B-fibers
Intermediate caliber, myelinated nerve fibers.

Bicuculline
GABA receptor antagonist.

Bradycardia
Abnormally slow heartbeat, usually defined as less than 60 beats per minute.

Callosotomy (also Corpus callosotomy)
Surgical procedure in which the corpus callosum is partially sectioned. Used as a treatment for atonic seizures.

Cardiac branches of the vagus nerve
Nerve fibers within the vagus nerve that innervate the heart.

Carotid sheath
Fibrous sheath around the carotid arteries and associated structures.

Carotid sinus
A slight dilation of the common carotid artery at its bifurcation, the walls of which are innervated by the intercarotid or sinus branch of the glossopharyngeal nerve. Concerned with the regulation of systemic blood pressure; when stimulated, there is a reflex slowing of the heart and vasodilation.

Centromedian nucleus (thalamus)
A mass of cells in the medial part of the thalamus lying lateral to the medial and posterior ventral nuclei and partly embedded in the internal medullary lamina.

C-fibers
Narrow-caliber, unmyelinated nerve fibers.

C fos, *see* Fos.

Cheyne-Stokes respiration
A particular cyclical breathing pattern characterized by a gradual increase in tidal volume followed by a progressive decline in tidal volume ending in apnea.

Complex partial seizures
Epileptic seizures arising from focal or localized region(s) of cortex that interrupt consciousness.

Corpus callosotomy, *see* Callosotomy.

Current (also Output current)
Amount of electrical current delivered in a single pulse of a stimulation; measured in milliamperes (mA).

Desynchronization
A pattern of the electroencephalogram in which anatomically related brain regions manifest rhythms that are different in frequency and/ or morphology.

Dorsal motor nucleus
A column of cells in the medulla oblongata in the floor of the fourth ventricle that gives rise to preganglionic parasympathetic fibers of the vagus nerve.

Double-blind
A study design in which neither the subject

nor the investigator knows which kind of treatment is being given until after the trial.

Duration, *see* Pulse duration.

Dysphagia
An abnormality of swallowing.

Dyspnea
Shortness of breath.

Epilepsy
Term used to describe all pathological states or diseases that are characterized by recurrent epileptic seizures. Epileptic seizures, in turn, are characterized by sudden, transient changes in the sensory system, the motor system, subjective well-being, and/ or behavior caused by a sudden, excessive, rapid discharge of the cortex of the brain.

Epileptic encephalopathy
Term used to describe epilepsy syndromes usually starting in early childhood and characterized by several types of seizures, markedly abnormal EEG background and cognitive dysfunction.

Ethanolamine
Cell membrane phospholipid precursor formed by the reduction of glycine or decarboxylation of serine.

Fos (also C Fos)

A nuclear protein signaling gene transcription; its expression is used as a functional marker for neurons that become activated under controlled experimental conditions.

Frequency *see* Stimulation frequency

Functional magnetic resonance imaging (fMRI)
Radiographic technique that identifies brain regions that are activated during cognitive, sensory and other tasks.

Gamma-amino butyric acid
GABA; the primary inhibitory neurotransmitter in the central nervous system.

Generalized-onset seizures
Seizures that originate from widespread, bilateral, cortical regions. Subtypes include tonic-clonic, tonic, clonic, atonic, myoclonic and absence seizures.

Generator, *see* Pulse generator.

Glutamate
Primary excitatory neurotransmitter in the central nervous system; precursor to GABA.

Helical coil
Configuration at the rostral end of the lead that allows the lead to nontraumatically adapt to the shape of the vagus nerve while ensuring

that the middle coil (with the platinum ribbon that conveys the electrical signal to the nerve) maintains optimum mechanical contact with the nerve.

Holter monitor
Diagnostic test in which heart rhythms are monitored for a prolonged period, typically 24 hours. Used to correlate episodic symptoms with simultaneous heart rhythms.

Horner's syndrome
Combination of ptosis, meiosis and anhydrosis due to a lesion affecting the cervical sympathetic nerve fibers.

Hypersynchronization
A pattern of the electroencephalogram in which anatomically related brain regions manifest rhythms that are similar in frequency and/or morphology.

Interrogation
The diagnostic process of determining whether there are any problems with wand-generator communications, lead impedance or the programmed current.

Kindling
An experimental model of epilepsy in which repeated subconvulsive electrical or chemical stimulations eventually induce a range of spontaneous behavioral seizures.

Lead
Stimulating electrode that transmits the electrical signal from the generator to the vagus nerve.

Lead test, see Interrogation.

Lennox-Gastaut Syndrome
A severe form of difficult-to-treat epilepsy characterized by multiple seizure types, cognitive dysfunction and markedly abnormal electroencephalogram.

Locus coeruleus
Collection of dorsal pontine neurons that provides extremely widespread noradrenergic innervation of the cortex, diencephalons and other brain structures. Derives its name from its bluish pigmented cells.

Magnet mode
The set of stimulation parameters that are programmed to be delivered upon placement of the magnet cover over the pulse generator.

Maximal electroshock
A particular model of experimental seizures in which an electrical stimulus is administered via corneal electrodes to an animal. Identifies compounds that prevent seizure spread.

Medulla oblongata
The most caudal section of the brainstem; critical for cardiac and respiratory function.

NeuroCybernetic Prosthesis®
Former name of VNS Therapy Pulse Generator. FDA-approved vagus nerve stimulation device for epilepsy.

Norepinephrine
A neurotransmitter produced by noradrenergic neurons and characteristic of the sympathetic nervous system.

Nucleus ambiguus
A column of cells in the lateral reticular formation; gives rise to efferent fibers of the glossopharyngeal, vagus and accessory nerves.

Nucleus prepositus hypoglossi
A group of cells extending from the hypoglossal nucleus to the caudal limit of the abducent nucleus. Synapses of this nucleus are inhibitory.

Nucleus of the spinal tract of the trigeminal nerve
The column of cells lying along the length of the spinal tract of the trigeminal nerve; receives terminations of the trigeminal nerve.

Nucleus of the tractus solitarius
The column of cells in the medulla near the solitary tract; receives terminations of the solitary tract.

Off time, see Signal off time.

On-demand stimulation
Transient change from the automatic

intermittent stimulation. May be brought on by the patient or a carer through placement of the supplied magnet on the patient's chest over the generator for several seconds. If the magnet is removed, automatic stimulation will resume.

On time, *see* Signal on time

Open-label (also Unblinded)
Refers to study design in which both the subject and the treating physician know the nature of the experimental treatment.

Output current, *see* Current.

Parabrachial nucleus
Cells of pontine origin that project to the nucleus tractus solitarius, the area postrema, the ventrolateral medulla and the periaqueductal gray.

Paresthesia
Numbness, tingling.

Partial-onset seizures
Seizures that arise and remain confined to a localized region of cortex.

Pentylenetetrazol
A convulsant used in an animal model of seizures identifying compounds that raise the seizure threshold.

Periaqueductal gray
Region of gray matter that encircles the cerebral aqueduct; involved in a variety of behaviors.

Pharmacoresistant epilepsy
Epileptic seizures that do not respond to pharmacotherapy (antiseizure medications). Also referred to as refractory, intractable or treatment-resistant epilepsy.

Pharmacotherapy
Refers to the use of drugs or pharmaceuticals for the treatment of a disorder or medical condition.

Phrenic nerve
Peripheral nerve that originates in the cervical spinal cord; innervates the diaphragm.

Positron emission tomography (PET)
Technique for mapping brain function that measures glucose metabolism.

Pulse duration, *see* Pulse width

Pulse generator
Programmable signal generator implanted in the patient's left upper chest. An antenna inside the generator receives programming radiofrequency signals from the telemetry (programming) wand and then transfers these signals to a microprocessor within the generator, thereby controlling the programmable stimulation variables.

Pulse width
The duration of a single pulse within a period of stimulation; expressed in microseconds.

Radiofrequency
Method of wireless communication between the telemetry wand and the pulse generator.

Ramp-up procedure
Adjustment of current to tolerance over several weeks after implantation.

Randomized trial
A study design in which the patient is randomly allocated to one of several treatment arms. Randomization reduces the bias of treatment assignment.

Raphe nuclei
Small neurons along the midline reticular formation from the medulla through the midbrain providing serotonergic innervation to widespread brain regions.

Refractory, *see* Pharmacoresistant epilepsy

Responder rate
Percentage of patients with at least 50% seizure reduction per 28 days of treatment compared to baseline.

Serotonin
Hydroxytryptamine; a neurotransmitter in the central nervous system derived from tryptophan and metabolized to 5-HIAA. Raising serotonin concentrations is a major principle in the treatment of depression.

Signal off time
The time interval between periods of stimulation; measured in seconds to minutes.

Signal on time
The length of time that output current is delivered; measured in seconds.

Signal width, *see* Pulse width

Single-blind
A study design in which the subject does not know which kind of treatment is being given until after the trial is over. The investigator is aware which treatment the subject receives.

Sinoatrial node
Cardiac source of electrical impulses that control heart function and rate.

Sternocleidomastoid muscle
Neck muscle that flexes and rotates the head.

Stimulation frequency
The number of single pulses of stimulation delivered per second; expressed in hertz.

Telemetry wand
Hand-held device that uses radiofrequency signals to communicate noninvasively with

the generator. The wand is powered by batteries and is connected to a compatible computer; software allows the programmer (e.g. physician) to adjust any of the programmable functions of the generator as clinically indicated.

Tolerance
Failure to maintain the therapeutic effect during long-term treatment.

Tonic-clonic seizures
A subtype of generalized seizures, previously called grand mal seizures.

Tunneling tool
Device used during surgery to advance the lead subcutaneously from the generator to the vagus nerve during the implantation procedure.

Vagus nerve
The tenth cranial nerve, which is composed of somatic and visceral afferents and efferents. Vagal afferents, which comprise 80% of all vagal fibers, arise from the lungs, aorta, heart and gastrointestinal tract, and travel to the brainstem. Most fibers synapse in the nucleus of the solitary tract; a small percentage project into the medullary medial reticular formation, cerebellum and nucleus cuneatus. The nucleus of the solitary tract in turn projects into many

regions, including the hypothalamus, amygdala, dorsal raphe, nucleus ambiguus, dorsal motor nucleus of the vagus, parabrachial nucleus and the thalamus, which projects into the insular cortex.

Special visceral efferents innervate the larynx and pharynx. The general visceral efferents provide parasympathetic innervation of the heart (resulting in slowing of the heart rate), lungs (bronchial constriction and pulmonary secretions) and gastrointestinal tract (increased peristalis and secretions).

Vagus nerve stimulation
Programmable stimulation of the cervical portion of the left vagus nerve through implanted electrodes under the control of a pulse generator which is typically implanted in the upper left chest.

Vasodepressor response
The reaction to a stimulus that results in a lowering of the blood pressure.

Video stroboscopy
Procedure used to visualize the vocal cords.

VNS
Abbreviation for vagus nerve stimulation (also called vagal nerve stimulation).

Wand, *see* telemetry wand.

Index